Managing Diabetes

FAST-TRACK

by Joan Clark-Warner, MS, RD, CDE

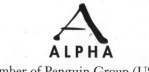

ALPHA

A member of Penguin Group (USA) Inc.

ALPHA BOOKS

Published by Penguin Group (USA) Inc.

Penguin Group (USA) Inc., 375 Hudson Street, New York, New York 10014, USA • Penguin
Group (Canada), 90 Eglinton Avenue East, Suite 700, Toronto, Ontario M4P 2Y3, Canada (a
division of Pearson Penguin Canada Inc.) • Penguin Books Ltd., 80 Strand, London WC2R 0RL,
England • Penguin Ireland, 25 St. Stephen's Green, Dublin 2, Ireland (a division of Penguin Books
Ltd.) • Penguin Group (Australia), 250 Camberwell Road, Camberwell, Victoria 3124, Australia (a
division of Pearson Australia Group Pty. Ltd.) • Penguin Books India Pvt. Ltd., 11 Community Centre,
Panchsheel Park, New Delhi—110 017, India • Penguin Group (NZ), 67 Apollo Drive, Rosedale,
North Shore, Auckland 1311, New Zealand (a division of Pearson New Zealand Ltd.) • Penguin Books
(South Africa) (Pty.) Ltd., 24 Sturdee Avenue, Rosebank, Johannesburg 2196, South Africa • Penguin
Books Ltd., Registered Offices: 80 Strand, London WC2R 0RL, England

Copyright © 2013 by Joan Clark-Warner, MS, RD, CDE

International Standard Book Number: 978-1-61564-244-1
Library of Congress Catalog Card Number: 2012947179

15 14 13   8 7 6 5 4 3 2 1

Interpretation of the printing code: The rightmost number of the first series of numbers is the year of
the book's printing; the rightmost number of the second series of numbers is the number of the book's
printing. For example, a printing code of 13-1 shows that the first printing occurred in 2013.

Printed in the United States of America

Note: This publication contains the opinions and ideas of its author. It is intended to provide helpful
and informative material on the subject matter covered. It is sold with the understanding that the author
and publisher are not engaged in rendering professional services in the book. If the reader requires
personal assistance or advice, a competent professional should be consulted.

The author and publisher specifically disclaim any responsibility for any liability, loss, or risk, personal or
otherwise, which is incurred as a consequence, directly or indirectly, of the use and application of any of
the contents of this book.

Most Alpha books are available at special quantity discounts for bulk purchases for sales promotions,
premiums, fund-raising, or educational use. Special books, or book excerpts, can also be created to fit
specific needs. For details, write: Special Markets, Alpha Books, 375 Hudson Street, New York, NY
10014.

Publisher: *Mike Sanders*	**Cover Designer:** *William Thomas*
Executive Managing Editor: *Billy Fields*	**Book Designers:** *William Thomas,*
Senior Acquisitions Editor: *Brook Farling*	*Rebecca Batchelor*
Development Editor: *Lynn Northrup*	**Indexer:** *Johnna Vanhoose Dinse*
Senior Production Editor: *Janette Lynn*	**Layout:** *Ayanna Lacey*
Copy Editor: *Amy Borrelli*	**Proofreader:** *Monica Stone*

Dedicated to my children, Tricia, Ryan, and Jenny; and their father, David.

Contents

Introduction

If you just found out that you have diabetes, you may be feeling confused, alone, and even terrified by what is happening to your body. You may wonder what kind of a life you will have going forward, and whether you can gain control over your diabetes. As a diabetes educator and gestational diabetic, I can tell you from experience that you can control your diabetes and maintain a great quality of life.

Here's a new twist on an old adage: "One step back, two steps forward." We learn from difficulties that arise in our lives. Maybe with diabetes we're learning that it's the little things in life that are really important, or perhaps we are learning how precious life is. Now is the time for you to take a step forward and learn how precious your life is. Your key to enjoying a full life and feeling better is to learn more about your diabetes.

In *The Complete Idiot's Guide to Managing Diabetes Fast-Track*, you will find the tools you need to stay healthy. This book contains important and updated information on how to care for your diabetes and health in a concise and practical way.

How This Book Is Organized

This book is divided into 10 chapters:

Chapter 1, Defining the Problem, defines diabetes and how to recognize its symptoms. You will learn about the three major types of diabetes and how to treat them. You will also learn about the complications that can occur with diabetes and the risk factors involved.

Chapter 2, Pillars of Managing Diabetes, explains the four approaches to managing diabetes: exercise, medications, diet, and a healthy lifestyle. Included will be an introduction to the diabetes health-care team and explanation of what each medical specialist can offer you in order to get optimal care.

Chapter 3, Medications and Monitoring, provides you with a guide to the best diabetic medications to use in order to avoid complications. It also shows you how to coordinate your medications with diet, how to prevent a low blood sugar, and, what to do if you get a low blood sugar.

Chapter 4, Eating to Control Blood Sugar, illustrates healthy ways to eat while controlling blood sugar. It also talks about the three basic nutrients in food and their impact on your blood sugar. Finally, it provides you with three major meal planning methods.

Chapter 5, Using the Glycemic Index, demonstrates how the glycemic index can be used to control your blood sugar, appetite, and weight status. It also provides you with proven ways to incorporate the GI into your diet.

Chapter 6, Weight Management and Diabetes, provides you with the tools to determine your calorie needs for weight loss or weight maintenance, and for monitoring your calorie intake. It also shows you what to look for when reading a label, and how to adjust insulin with a decreased calorie and carbohydrate intake. Finally, this chapter provides diabetic- and weight-savvy menus to help get you started.

Chapter 7, Strategies for Healthy Eating, provides you with step-by-step methods of changing and maintaining healthy eating habits. Included are tips for rearranging work and home environments, suggestions on visualizing your goals, and how to dine out and attend social eating functions without gaining weight.

Chapter 8, Exercise and Diabetes, teaches you how to exercise while taking insulin and insulin-secreting medications, and what to eat and drink prior to exercise.

Chapter 9, Supplements for Diabetes, helps you decide whether you need supplements, and tells you which vitamins, minerals, spices, and fiber supplements can potentially lower your blood sugar levels. Finally, it shows you what anti-inflammatory and antioxidant supplements you can use to your benefit.

Chapter 10, Special Beverages, Condiments, and Foods, contains information on how some diabetic convenience foods can help to make planning easy. It also shows you how to obtain quality packaged foods. Finally, it provides guidelines for use of sugar substitutes, salt, diet soda, alcohol, and coffee.

Extras

There is a lot of information to learn about caring for diabetes. To help you along, look for special tip, definition, and caution sidebars sprinkled throughout the book:

TO YOUR HEALTH

These tips will help you keep feeling your best.

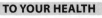
DEFINITION

Enhance your understanding of diabetes with these definitions.

RED FLAG

Be careful! Protect yourself from short- and long-term complications.

Acknowledgments

I'd like to thank my husband, Douglas, for his emotional support and editing assistance, and his patience while I was unavailable for several months while writing this book.

Special thanks to my boss, Laura, who provided emotional support and extra time off to complete this book; and to my family, clients, co-workers, and friends who have inspired me along the way.

Special thanks to my children, Jenny, Ryan, and Tricia, for their inspiration, enthusiasm, and creativity.

Special thanks to copy editor Amy Borrelli, senior production editor Janette Lynn, and technical editor Linda Griffen.

Finally, special thanks to Marilyn Allen of Allen O'Shea Literary Agency and Brook Farling of Alpha Books for their expertise and guidance in writing this book, and to development editor Lynn Northrup for her insights and processing guidance.

Special Thanks to the Technical Reviewer

The Complete Idiot's Guide to Managing Diabetes Fast-Track was reviewed by an expert who double-checked the accuracy of what you'll learn here, to help us ensure that this book gives you everything you need to know about managing your diabetes. Special thanks are extended to Linda Griffen.

Linda Griffen, BA, has been a Certified Clinical Research Coordinator and Research Associate at the University of Utah since 1978, focusing on epidemiology, hematology/oncology, endocrinology, and urogynecology.

Trademarks

All terms mentioned in this book that are known to be or are suspected of being trademarks or service marks have been appropriately capitalized. Alpha Books and Penguin Group (USA) Inc. cannot attest to the accuracy of this information. Use of a term in this book should not be regarded as affecting the validity of any trademark or service mark.

Defining the Problem

Annie felt upset as she walked out of her doctor's office. A storm of emotions washed through her. She felt angry, then sad, then anxious. She thought, "There must be some mistake, I can't have diabetes! Maybe they got my test mixed up with someone else's."

Unfortunately for Annie, it was her third positive test. Annie had diabetes!

Like Annie, you might have been told you have diabetes and are finding it hard to believe. You may not be able to make your diabetes go away, but there are steps you can take to either manage your symptoms or eliminate diabetes altogether. If you eliminate symptoms, you are no longer considered diabetic. If you have prediabetes or a mild type 2 diabetes, your chances of eliminating your diabetes will be higher. To learn how to manage and perhaps eliminate symptoms, you will need to know more about the type of diabetes you have, its related conditions, and how these conditions can affect you. This chapter will help.

What Is Diabetes?

Diabetes is a condition where the body either does not produce enough insulin or is unable to use the insulin that it makes. Without insulin, your cells cannot use the energy from your food well or at all.

When you eat, the food is broken down into basic substances that your body can use for energy. One of these substances is glucose (also called blood sugar), which is the form of sugar that is used by your cells for energy.

Insulin is crucial in helping your body move your blood sugar into your cells. If blood sugar can't enter the cells, it will build up in the blood. This condition is a disorder called diabetes.

There are three major types of diabetes: type 1, type 2, and gestational. Many of the symptoms of the different types of diabetes are the same; however, it's the causes that make each type different.

Type 1 Diabetes

Type 1 diabetes accounts for about 9 percent of diabetics. It is an *autoimmune* condition that generally occurs in childhood and adolescence. People with type 1 diabetes can't make their own insulin, so they need to take it. Without insulin your body can't absorb the energy (calories) and nutrients you need to survive, and without adequate calorie absorption you lose weight. Consequently, if you have this type of diabetes, you are probably on the thin side. When you start taking insulin you will regain some of weight you lost.

Insulin injections are usually taken from a 10 ml vial. A needle attached to a syringe is inserted into the vial to extract a specific amount of insulin. The needle is then removed from the vial and flicked to remove any air bubbles prior to injecting its contents into specific fat areas on the body. If you have to do this, you will be shown how by your health care providers.

DEFINITION

An **autoimmune** condition occurs when the body fails to recognize its own body parts as "self" and so allows its immune response (antibodies) to attack those parts.

Beta Cells and Diagnosis

Insulin normally comes from cells in the pancreas called beta cells. With type 1 diabetes, these cells no longer function. In addition to the beta cells, the pancreas has ductal and acinar cells that make digestive enzymes. A person with type 1 diabetes can usually make digestive enzymes.

When you are initially diagnosed, your doctor will run an antibody blood test to determine what type of diabetes you have. Type 1 diabetics make antibodies that attack their beta cells.

Ketoacidosis

Type 1 diabetics who do not make insulin and type 2 diabetics who do not make enough insulin can experience very high blood glucose levels. They could even end up with a life-threatening condition called diabetic *ketoacidosis*.

DEFINITION

Ketoacidosis is a condition in which elevated blood glucose levels cause severe dehydration and loss of important electrolytes (minerals such as potassium and magnesium). If not treated, confusion, decreased ability to breathe, increased heart rate, and sometimes a heart attack can occur.

Treatment and Risk

There are several types of insulin that can be used if you can't make insulin or enough insulin. These insulin types and their uses are listed in Chapter 3, which discusses medication.

The risk of developing type 1 diabetes for someone with no family history of it is low. If someone in your family has type 1 diabetes, your chances of developing it are slightly higher. However, even if you are more genetically prone to type 1 diabetes, there is usually an environmental incident that also needs to be present to trigger it. Some research suggests that environmental triggers could include drinking too much cow's milk as a child or contracting a virus at a young age.

Gestational Diabetes

Gestatational diabetes occurs in up to 3 percent of all pregnancies and has a significant genetic component. The growing fetus and placenta's secreting hormones decrease the body's sensitivity to insulin, which leads to increased blood glucose levels.

Diagnosis

Gestational diabetes is diagnosed by an abnormal OGTT (oral glucose tolerance test). For the test you will be asked to fast for eight hours. Then you will drink a liquid that contains between 75 and 100 grams of glucose (a easy-to-digest carbohydrate). About 23 sugar packets make 100 grams of glucose, so this drink will taste very sweet and syrupy. In this form and at this amount a high demand is placed on the body to produce an adequate amount of insulin. It is not typical of the amount or type of carbohydrate that is normally consumed in a meal.

A sample of your blood will be taken before you do this test and then again at 30- to 60-minute intervals. The test takes three hours to complete. In a normal situation the blood sugar increases to its highest point in approximately one hour, then it starts on its way back down to a base level. The usual target numbers vary depending on whether the blood sugar is measured after drinking an almost pure glucose solution versus eating a meal.

Normal blood values for a 100-gram oral glucose tolerance test are as follows:

- Fasting (the blood sugar taken at least eight hours after eating): <95
- One hour after eating: <190
- Two hours after eating: <155
- Three hours after eating: <140

If you compare pregnancy blood sugar levels to a nonpregnant person, you will find the blood sugar is naturally lower during pregnancy. Average blood sugar in pregnant women without gestational diabetes are at these levels when eating a typical meal such as chicken, vegetables, yogurt, and a potato.:

- Fasting: 71 (+/-8)
- One hour after meal: 109 (+/-13)
- Two hours after meal: 99 (+/-10)

Treatment

A special diet, oral medication, or insulin may be needed during the duration of the pregnancy. Blood sugar control is especially important in pregnancy. When the fetus is exposed to high levels of sugar, there are significant changes in the way its genes are expressed, and this can affect the baby for the rest of its life. In addition, high blood sugar tends to make babies larger, which can cause problems at the time of delivery.

RED FLAG

If you have gestational diabetes, you will be happy to know that your blood sugar will return to normal levels after childbirth. However, your chances of having gestational diabetes in future pregnancies is increased, and your risk of developing diabetes later in life will also be higher, especially if you are over 30 years old, overweight, or inactive.

Type 2 Diabetes

Like gestational diabetes, type 2 diabetes is often genetic, and is more pronounced if you are obese, have an inactive lifestyle, poor eating habits, or are older. Type 2 diabetes makes up more than 90 percent of all diabetics.

Insulin Resistance

If you have type 2 diabetes, you produce some insulin, but your cells cannot produce enough insulin, or they are unable to use the insulin efficiently. The condition in which insulin can't be used efficiently is called insulin resistance. People are not born with insulin resistance but can become this way by gaining too much weight or not exercising enough.

Initially, a person with insulin resistance can compensate by making extra insulin. This keeps their blood sugar in check. After years of overproducing insulin, the beta cells in the pancreas can wear out. When the pancreas wears out, it stops making enough insulin, and blood glucose levels abnormally increase.

Diagnosis

People with type 2 diabetes will have any of the following blood sugar levels:

- A fasting blood sugar ≥126
- A blood sugar taken anytime ≥200
- Two-hours-after-meal blood sugar ≥200
- An *HbgA1C* test ≥6.5 percent

> **DEFINITION**
>
> An **HbgA1C** test measures the amount of glucose that gets bound to hemoglobin (red blood cells) over a two- to three-month period. Glucose that enters the blood "sugarcoats" the red blood cells. The more glucose in the blood, the more the hemoglobin gets sugarcoated.

More explanations for these tests can be found in Chapter 3 on monitoring.

Treatment and Risk

Depending on the severity of your condition, type 2 diabetes may be treated with diet only, with oral diabetic medications along with diet, and/or with insulin. Diabetic medication and their uses are described in Chapter 3.

Being overweight is the strongest acquired risk factor for type 2 diabetes. A large portion of this book will show you how to deal with excess body weight in order to help decrease the symptoms of diabetes.

Prediabetes

In this condition, blood sugar is beginning to show increases but is not yet high enough to be considered diabetes. Studies have shown that by keeping blood sugar levels within normal limits and your weight at a healthy level you may be able to get rid of your pre-diabetes and avoid developing type 2 diabetes. This may mean losing weight, increasing activity, and following your doctor's instructions to remain in good health.

Diagnosis

Prediabetes is diagnosed when there is an *impaired fasting glucose (IFG)* or *impaired glucose intolerance (IGT)*. To determine the fasting glucose, the individual does not eat for 8 to 12 hours. To determine if an individual has an impaired glucose tolerance, a glucose-rich drink, as described earlier for gestational diabetes testing, is taken and the blood sugar values tested one and two hours afterward.

📖 **DEFINITION**

Impaired fasting glucose (IFG) is a condition in which the fasting blood glucose level is elevated above what is considered normal, but not high enough to be considered type 2 diabetes. **Impaired glucose intolerance (IGT)** is a condition in which the increase in blood glucose that occurs after consuming 75 g of glucose is greater than normal, but not high enough as in people with type 2 diabetes.

Following are normal and impaired fasting and two-hours-after-meal glucose levels:

- Normal fasting glucose: 80 to 120
- Normal two hours after glucose drink: <140
- IFG (impaired fasting glucose): 100 to 125
- IGT (impaired glucose tolerance) two hours after glucose drink: >140

Treatment and Risk

Prediabetes is a serious condition. Research shows that some long-term damage can be done to the heart and circulatory system during prediabetes. However, by taking steps to prevent the onset of type 2 diabetes, you can decrease the risk of damage. Changes such as maintaining a healthy weight, eating healthy, and exercise can return your blood sugar to the normal range again. If you do not improve with diet and exercise alone, oral medication may also be used to help keep your blood sugar within a normal range.

If you have diabetes or prediabetes, your doctor may have given you a blood glucose meter so that you can regularly test your blood glucose levels.

Symptoms

Elevated blood glucose levels can cause symptoms. If you experience any of the following conditions, your blood sugar is most likely elevated:

- Frequent urination
- Unusual thirst
- Frequent infections
- Blurred vision
- Wounds that do not heal well
- Tingling or numbness in the feet or hands
- Unusual irritability
- Unusual fatigue

Although it is common to experience some of these symptoms, some type 2 diabetic and prediabetic people report that they have no symptoms.

Metabolic Syndrome

Many type 2 diabetics start out not only with prediabetes, but have what is called metabolic syndrome, with symptoms including insulin resistance, weight gain, abdominal fat, high blood pressure, a high triglyceride level, and a low HDL ("good cholesterol") level. The following levels are used to determine this syndrome:

- Abdominal obesity: a waist circumference ≥40 inches for men and ≥35 inches for women
- Elevated fasting serum triglyceride levels: ≥150
- Low serum HDL: ≤40 in men and ≤50 in women
- Hypertension or high blood pressure: ≥130/85
- Fasting blood sugar: ≥100

A person with metabolic syndrome has three or more of these five symptoms. Research shows that when a group of these symptoms occur together, more health complications can occur than if they occur separately.

RED FLAG

According to research done in 2010 by the Centers for Disease Control and Prevention (CDC), people with metabolic syndrome are five times more likely to develop diabetes and three times more likely to develop cardiovascular disease than those who do not have metabolic syndrome.

If you have metabolic syndrome and can correct some of these symptoms, you can decrease your risk of complications. This is especially true if you lose weight. (I'll discuss weight management in Chapter 6.)

Complications and Risks of Diabetes and Prediabetes

Even if you feel fine now, it is never a good idea to become careless with your health. This is especially true when you have diabetes or are at an increased risk for diabetes. Damage caused by high blood sugar levels can go unnoticed until it is too late.

Complications

Cardiologists who perform heart transplants understand their patients are often at higher risk of dying younger from complications. What we now know is that there is an underlying reason for these young deaths. More than half of cardiovascular patients have diabetes or prediabetes, and more than 75 percent are overweight. Diabetes, prediabetes, and overweight conditions are seen in many cardiovascular units across the country.

Elevated blood glucose, insulin resistance, and obesity increase inflammation and *dyslipidemia*. Over time, dyslipidemia can lead to *atherosclerosis* and cause blockage. These blockages deprive tissues of oxygen. When heart and brain tissue cannot get oxygen, the result is a heart attack or a stroke.

> **DEFINITION**
>
> **Dyslipidemia** refers to abnormal amounts of lipids (fats) in the blood. **Atherosclerosis,** also called hardening of the arteries, is a common disorder in which fat, cholesterol, and other substances build up on the walls of the arteries.

In addition to cardiovascular disease, other complications of poorly controlled diabetes and prediabetes include the following conditions:

* Poor eyesight, light sensitivity, night blindness, or blindness.
* Poor circulation, leads to feet, hands, and leg injuries that won't heal as expected.
* Stroke. It is estimated that 37 to 42 percent of all ischemic (constricted vein) strokes are due to the effects of diabetes.
* Nerve damage leading to pain, tingling, and loss of feeling in extremities.
* Problems digesting food, resulting in bloating, gas, indigestion, or gastroparesis (slow emptying of the stomach).
* Erectile dysfunction in men.
* Kidney damage. According to the National Kidney Foundation, approximately 44 percent of kidney failure is caused by diabetes.

Remember, to avoid these complications and possible surgery, use an aggressive approach in resolving your elevated blood glucose levels. When you use more prevention in your everyday diabetes care, you increase your quality of life and limit your complications.

Risk Factors

If you have some risk factors for diabetes you already know about, you may wonder if anything you can do will really make a difference. Despite your genes, there are things you can do to make a positive change in your health. Here are some of the risk factors that can cause complications with diabetes. Some of these factors, like age and ethnic background, you can't do anything about, but you can make a difference by making changes in your diet, lifestyle, and weight:

- A family history of diabetes
- An age greater than 45 years
- Prior gestational diabetes
- Excess body weight, especially around the waist
- Metabolic syndrome
- Lifestyle with a low activity level
- Having given birth to a baby weighing more than 9 pounds
- HDL cholesterol of <35 mg/dL
- Triglyceride levels of ≥250 mg/dL
- Ethnicity (African Americans, Mexican Americans, American Indians, native Hawaiians, and some Asian Americans have increased risk of diabetes)
- Skipping meals and overeating at other meals
- Eating too many calories (especially in simple carbohydrates) and not enough fiber
- Chronic psychological stress
- Sleep deprivation

Number-One Risk Factor: Obesity

Obesity is the strongest acquired risk factor for type 2 diabetes. It is estimated that one out of every three adults in the United States is overweight. In addition, the CDC projects that by 2030, 42 percent of the population will be obese. Despite these statistics, you are a step ahead of the general population. You have taken action to improve your condition by reading this book. Good! You can and will improve your diabetes with guidance and personal commitment.

Are you overweight? If you decide you want to lose weight, the chapters that follow on diet, weight management, and exercise will help you. You can determine your ideal body weight (IBW) using an easy formula developed by research physician Dr. Carol Ireton-Jones. The formula was derived from statistics of healthy populations with the lowest death rates. Here it is:

- **Women:** IBW = 100 pounds for the first 60 inches in height, then add an extra 5 pounds for every inch over 60 inches. For example, here's the calculation for a woman with a height of 65 inches:

  60 inches = 100 lbs

  5 inches × 5 = 25 lbs

  IBW = 100 lbs + 25 lbs = 125 lbs (+/-10 percent)

- **Men:** IBW = 106 pounds for the first 60 inches in height, then add an extra 6 pounds for every inch over 60 inches. For example, here's the calculation for a man with a height of 72 inches:

  60 inches = 106 lbs

  12 inches × 6 = 72 lbs

  IBW = 106 lbs + 72 lbs = 178 lbs (+/-10 percent)

This formula can also account for bone structure by using a weight range of plus or minus 10 percent. If you have smaller bone structure you will be at the bottom of your IBW range. Conversely, if you have larger bone structure, you will be at the top of your IBW range.

If, after calculating your IBW, you find you are a little heavier than you would like to be, don't despair. Know that even a small amount of weight loss can significantly increase insulin sensitivity. With better insulin sensitivity you will not need as much medication and/or insulin, and less medication and insulin can in turn result in even great weight loss. This is because some diabetic medications and insulin can actually cause weight gain. You will find out more about what diabetic medications are best in Chapter 3, and find weight management diet strategies in Chapters 5, 6, and 7.

Pillars of Managing Diabetes

Mary yawned and thought, "Why am I so tired all the time? I'm only 42, this shouldn't be happening! Maybe if I lost some weight it would help." She then decided to call her friend Jane for some emotional support.

"Hi, Jane! Do you want to go on a weight-loss diet with me?"

"Okay, but I'm a little concerned," Jane replied. Last time we tried to diet, we ate even more than we usually do."

"Yeah, I know, but I'm just so hungry all the time," Mary conceded.

"What about going to see your doctor for a checkup before you start weight loss? You might have some kind of metabolism problem. Also, remember last week, you told me that you were having tingling and numbness in your feet? If you go see a doctor, tell him about that, too."

Two days later, Mary made an appointment with her doctor. After a thorough examination he told her that she had type 2 diabetes. He also referred her to an endocrinologist and a diabetes educator. They provided her with diabetic medication, a glucometer, and a diet especially designed for her.

This chapter will explain the multifaceted approaches used for managing diabetes and will introduce you to the health-care providers who are best equipped to help with your diabetes.

A Multifaceted Approach

Major approaches used to help manage diabetes include diet, physical activity, medication therapy, and a healthy lifestyle. Each approach is interactive and works best when coordinated. If you use a multifaceted approach, your health will greatly improve.

TO YOUR HEALTH

Exercise + medication therapy + diet + healthy lifestyle = a healthy you!

Exercise

Exercise has been shown to help prevent the complications of diabetes and increase longevity. It can also help control your diabetes by:

- Improving your body's use of insulin.
- Improving your mood.
- Burning excess body fat.
- Protecting against heart and blood vessel disease.
- Improving bone density.
- Increasing muscle strength.
- Increasing circulation.
- Reducing stress.
- Increasing overall energy level.

Before starting an exercise program, get an okay from your doctor, who may prohibit some types of exercise depending on your present condition. Consider getting additional help from an exercise trainer. To learn more about exercise and diabetes, see Chapter 8.

Medications

If you have type 2 diabetes or are prediabetic, you may not need medication. However, if diet and physical activity are not successful alone, medications can be added. These medications may be oral medications, noninsulin injections, and/or insulin. If you have type 1 diabetes, you will need to take insulin. Insulin can be provided by an insulin pump or by injections. As I'll discuss in Chapter 3, the right medication for the right condition is a must. To have medications prescribed for you, you must see a doctor, physician assistant, or nurse practitioner.

Diet

There are many studies that show the benefits of a diabetic diet in reducing and preventing complications such as eye, nerve, cardiovascular, and kidney disease. The diabetic diet focuses on foods with modified amounts of carbohydrates, healthy fats, high fiber, and unprocessed foods. Total calories are spread out evenly into three meals and a couple of snacks through the day. In addition, the diet can incorporate weight management. See Chapters 4, 5, and 6 for more details about diet.

To help you match medication and insulin to the right amount of carbohydrates, see a dietitian or a diabetes educator. The educator can help you improve your blood sugar, help prevent problems such as cardiovascular and kidney disease, and assist you in maintaining a healthy body weight. See the section "Working with Your Health-Care Team" later in this chapter to learn more.

A Healthy Lifestyle

A healthy lifestyle includes getting adequate rest, having a supportive family and/or friends, being involved in community activities, learning, and finding out how to cope with stress. Studies show that these attributes can keep you healthier and help control your blood sugar. See Chapter 7 for more details.

The health-care people who can help you with lifestyle changes include counselors, psychologists, psychiatrists, and social workers. Resources that can help you with behavior changes include community classes and support groups. Some of the topics discussed in the classes and support groups include carbohydrate counting, weight management, stress reduction, and diabetic medications. Check with your doctor to get started.

Working with Your Health-Care Team

To help you start implementing the multifaceted approach (medication, diet, exercise, and a healthy lifestyle), contact your doctor. He can refer you to the health-care providers who are best equipped to help with diabetes, including endocrinologists and certified diabetes educators (CDEs). These health care providers are your allies and support squad. Working with them will help you learn how to manage your diabetes.

Endocrinologist

An endocrinologist specializes in diseases that affect your glands (endocrine system). These glands include the thyroid, parathyroid, pancreas, ovaries, testes, adrenal, pituitary, and hypothalamus. The gland in the endocrine system that is most closely involved with diabetes is the pancreas.

Your endocrinologist will often perform a variety of tests requiring blood and/or urine samples. He will also check for signs of tissue or nerve damage, and check your vital signs (blood pressure, heart rate, breathing rate). These tests can help your endocrinologist determine the best course for your treatment.

An endocrinologist will refer you for diabetes education, for further tests you may need, and to other health care specialists. The referrals to see other health care team members such as a diabetes educator, a podiatrist, psychologist, or licensed clinical social worker are covered by most insurance carriers, including Medicare, as long as your diabetes condition has been diagnosed.

It is vital that you communicate with your endocrinologist. Provide him with all the information you have. Try to accurately describe your symptoms. Are you tired a lot, do you have indigestion, do you have numbness in any of your hands and feet, or do you have a wound that won't heal? Write down anything that is bothering you before your doctor visit so you can be sure to discuss it. It's helpful to keep a record of your blood sugar, which includes some morning fasting values and some values after meals, especially two hours after a meal. Be sure to take this to your appointment.

Your endocrinologist will determine if you need medication for your diabetes. He can decide on the best type of medication. Let him know what your personal goals are, such as losing weight. Some medications are helpful for weight management, some are not. If you have kidney disease in your family history, be sure to mention that. Some medications are helpful in the prevention of kidney disease. Make your concerns known.

 RED FLAG

Ask yourself if your doctor has shown a genuine interest in you. Do you feel good with him? If not, you may want to find a doctor whom you feel more comfortable with.

Certified Diabetes Educator

Certified diabetes educators have gone through rigorous training and testing and are required to stay current in their field in order to stay certified. Certified educators have the initials CDE (certified diabetes educator) after their name.

CDEs most often include nurses, doctors, dietitians, and pharmacists. Some other educators (not CDEs) teach only within specialized areas such as diet or medications. All CDEs, whether a dietitian, nurse, or pharmacist, are qualified to teach in all areas of diabetes care.

Here are just some important diabetes care skills that a CDE can teach you:

- How to monitor and take your blood sugar with a glucometer
- How to take your oral medications
- How to take insulin
- How to determine the right amount of insulin for a specific amount of carbohydrate consumed at a meal
- Treatments for low or high blood sugar when on insulin
- How to time medications with exercise
- How to count carbohydrate grams
- How to adjust insulin based on blood sugar
- How to prevent complications on sick days
- How to prevent foot damage

Visiting with the Diabetes Educator

In your first couple of appointments after being referred by your endocrinologist, you will most likely see a dietitian, nurse, or pharmacist diabetes educator in an office setting. No matter what educator you see, always bring a record of your blood glucose levels to the meeting. Your educator will teach you how to do this in order to provide the information you will need to learn about how you respond to food and for the educator to help you learn what to do.

Classes

Diabetes educators generally teach classes in addition to seeing people on a one-on-one basis. After your initial appointments, you may be asked to attend some diabetes classes. These classes consist of three or more diabetics at a time. They can be helpful and are cheaper because several people will share an educator's time. Insurance policies specify the number of individual or class visits allowed in your plan. Typical classes taught include the Basics of Diabetes, Carbohydrate Counting, Effective Monitoring, and Exercise with Diabetes. These classes both instruct and provide you with a support group.

> **TO YOUR HEALTH**
>
> Many insurance companies now cover diabetes education (both individual sessions and classes) if done by a CDE. The name used by insurance companies for diabetes training is called Diabetes Self-Management Training (DSMT). Coverage usually allows for 10 sessions. Each session can last for up to two hours.

Diabetes Educator Meetings

When you want to focus on your individual diet, you will see a dietitian/diabetes educator. She can help you design a diet tailored to meet your goals. Your diet may include weight management, meal planning and/or carbohydrate counting. Bring to the meeting a log of your typical food intake for one to three days and a list of the vitamins, minerals, and herbal supplements that you take.

When you want to focus on medications and their interactions, see a pharmacist/diabetes educator. Bring a list of all of your medications and vitamin-herbal supplements, as well as your blood glucose log to this meeting.

Other diabetic training topics include how to use an insulin pump, giving insulin injections, exercising with diabetes, or what to do on sick days. These topics are often taught by a nurse/ diabetes educator.

Whether you see a nurse, pharmacist, or dietitian, you will be provided with written educational materials and a glucometer (a meter to check your blood sugar at home). Diabetes educators should be able to answer most of your questions pertaining to diabetes, but if not, they have the authority to refer you to other specialists, such as a pharmacist or a social worker.

Other Health-Care Professionals

The risk of having eye, foot, and teeth/gum problems is higher if you have diabetes. In addition to seeing an endocrinologist and CDE, you might see an eye doctor (ophthalmologist) for a dilated eye exam annually or as needed, a foot doctor (podiatrist), and seek special attention to diabetes from your own dentist.

Eye Doctor

An ophthalmologist, unlike an optometrist, has a medical degree (MD) and has completed three to six years of specialized training. He will check your dilated eyes to see if any changes have occurred in the retina or other structures of the eye. If a problem is spotted, he can intervene to prevent further damage. If you have diabetes, see an ophthalmologist at least once a year.

Podiatrist

Foot conditions can occur with diabetes because of poor circulation, neuropathy (nerve damage), or poor blood glucose control. If you have neuropathy, you might not notice a cut or scrape on your foot. If left untreated, an injury can become severe enough to require amputation. Pay attention to even tiny injuries.

If you are not able to inspect your own feet and you have neu-ropathy, you should have someone you know check your feet regularly. In addition to checking the condition of your feet, it is wise to visit a podiatrist at least once a year. A podiatrist will determine if you have any foot or nail deformities or disease, which could create complications.

Dentist

A high blood sugar level can cause problems with your teeth and gums. Diabetes lowers your ability to resist infection and slows healing.

Gum disease is more common because high blood sugar make it harder to fight bacteria. Bacteria like sugar! As bacteria grow, more plaque can build up on your teeth. The longer plaque and tartar remain on your teeth, the more it can irritate your gums. After a while the gums become swollen and bleed easily. This is called gum disease or gingivitis. If gingivitis is left untreated, it can lead to a more serious infection called periodontitis. Periodontitis can destroy the soft tissue and bone that support your teeth. It can also cause your overall blood sugar level to rise, making the condition even harder to treat.

Preventing and treating gingivitis and periodontitis can help improve your blood sugar control. You should see your dentist every 3 to 6 months.

Preparing for Your Appointment

Be prepared for each of your appointments. Write down your questions prior to your visit. Ask your health-care provider enough questions to optimize your visit and to address your concerns. Think of anything that has been causing problems for you and write it down. Here are some specific questions that you might want to ask:

- What is causing my problems?
- What is my long-term outlook with and without treatment?

- How accurate are the tests for diagnosing my problem?
- When will I get my test results?
- What are my treatment options?
- What are my alternatives?
- What are the side effects of the medications that you are prescribing?
- Will this medication interact with my other medications?
- How do you spell the name of my medication?
- Are my medications called more than one name?

Electronic Learning

Learning about diabetes takes time and patience, but the more informed you become, the better able you will be to manage your health. In addition to visiting the health-care team and learning through others, you may want to go online. Here are some websites you might want to visit:

- American Diabetes Association: diabetes.org
- Academy of Nutrition and Dietetics: eatright.org/public
- Nutrient Data Base for Standard Reference: ndb.nal. usda.gov
- National Health Information Center: health.gov
- MyFoodAdvisor: tracker.diabetes.org/explore
- The Centers for Disease Control and Prevention: cdc.gov

Medications and Monitoring

Irene checked her blood sugar two hours after she had eaten and found it to be 200. "How could that be?" she asked. "I just ate my usual meal; it should be around 140, like usual." John, her husband, overheard her talking to herself from the other room and walked toward her. "Is this about that new medication you're taking, Irene?"

"Yes, I think so, John. I'll have to monitor my blood sugar and call my doctor."

Changes in medications may cause changes in expected blood sugar values. Irene is not the only diabetic to experience this type of change, but she was able to make some adjustments and improve her blood sugar readings because she had been monitoring them. Monitoring blood sugar levels is absolutely necessary when it comes to maintaining good blood sugar control.

If you have blood sugar problems, you need to learn how to manage them using the correct diabetic medications based on your goals. Furthermore, you need to learn how to avoid the complications that can occur with diabetes and diabetic medications.

Monitoring Blood Glucose

The three major approaches used to control blood sugar are diet, physical activity, and medication. However, in order for all these approaches to work effectively, it is important that you monitor your blood sugar levels.

Blood sugar testing provides useful information to keep your blood sugar in a healthy range. It can help you judge how you are doing with your blood sugar after eating, exercising, and during illness and times of stress. It's relatively painless to check your blood sugar levels. A short, needlelike device called a lancet is used to prick your finger to obtain a drop of blood. The blood drop is put into a portable electronic device called a glucometer or glucose meter. There are many different types of meters, but they all work in a similar fashion. You place the drop of blood on a test strip in the meter and read your blood sugar level. Your pharmacist, doctor, or nurse can demonstrate how to use a glucometer and suggest a type of meter for you. You may be provided a meter at your first education visit and instructed in its use at that first meeting.

TO YOUR HEALTH

Before you get a meter and test strips, ask your insurance company, Medicare, or Medicaid about coverage. Test strips and meters will often vary from one policy to another. With Medicare it is required by law to cover test strips, but only certain types will be covered.

Testing Times

The frequency of testing depends on whether you are taking insulin, if you are sick, or whether you have a medication change. Most diabetics should take a fasting blood sugar, which requires that at least eight hours have lapsed prior to the test. This blood sugar is usually taken in the morning before breakfast. Testing is also commonly done before meals. Other times might include taking the blood glucose two hours after a meal, before and after exercise, or any time when you don't feel well.

Blood Sugar Goals

Diabetic blood sugar goals can differ based upon the guidelines you want to follow and your doctor's recommendations. The American Diabetes Association blood glucose goals are more moderate, whereas the American Association of Endocrinologists has stricter goals. The strict glucose goal guidelines are often referred to as "tight" glucose control. See the following table to find both diabetic types of control as well as normal blood glucose levels. Both sets of values are important for different reasons, and your doctor will use the one best for you.

Hemoglobin A1C

In the table, you probably recognize the general blood sugar numbers, but you may not be familiar with the term Hemoglobin A1C (HbA1C). The HbA1C test is performed at your health-care clinic. It is a common blood test used to diagnose and evaluate the care of diabetes. Other words for HbA1C are glycated hemoglobin, glycosylated hemoglobin, or hemoglobin A1C. We will use A1C as the common term here. The test result reflects what your average blood sugar range is for the past two to three months. It measures what percent of your hemoglobin (a red blood cell protein) is coated with sugar (glycated). The higher your A1C, the worse your blood sugar control and the higher your risk of diabetic complications. If you have a high A1C, you will need to take medication to help control your blood sugar.

Nondiabetic and Diabetic Blood Sugar Goals

Blood Sugar Time	Nondiabetic Normal (mg/dL)	Diabetic Tight Control (mg/dL)	Diabetic Moderate Control (mg/dL)
Fasting	<100	70–120	70–130
Two hours after a meal	<140	≤140–160	≤180
HbA1CA1C	4-5.7%	≤6.5%	≤7%
Before eating	<100	<110	<130

Source: American Diabetes Association and Endocrine Society.

Medication Intervention

Managing diet and physical activity is sometimes all that is required to achieve glycemic (blood sugar) control. However, this is not always the case. An oral medication or insulin with the diet and exercise together may be needed for good blood sugar control. There are many safe diabetic medications to use. If you are a type 2 diabetic and are able to lose weight, you may eventually be able to decrease or discontinue your medication. Your first goal, however, is good blood sugar control.

Presently, diabetic medications can be taken by mouth or injected. Pharmaceutical companies have been working on other ways to administer insulin, including inhaled insulin, which was predicted to be on the market in 2010 but is still unavailable. This is because research shows that there may be a possible increased rate of lung cancer with its use.

Oral Medications

There are many oral diabetic medications. Some can help stimulate insulin production, others can help your own insulin to work better, and still others can retard carbohydrate absorption.

Oral diabetic medications are generally used for type 2 diabetes and prediabetes. There are six major categories of oral medications:

- Sulfonylureas
- Meglitinides
- Biguanides
- Thiazolidinediones
- Alpha-glucosidase inhibitors
- Dipeptidyl-peptidase-4 (DPP-4) inhibitors

The following table shows the specific medications within each of these categories and their effects. Your doctor will decide which is right for you and see that you are instructed in the reasons you are using your medication and how to use it. When you see your doctor in following visits, he will want to know your progress to see if this continues to be the best medication for you.

Action and Effects of Oral Medications Commonly Used for Diabetes

Class	Action and Effects	Medications (Generic Name)	Medications (Brand Name)
Sulfonylureas	Stimulates insulin secretion, may cause weight gain, long acting	Glipizide Glyburide Glimepiride	Glucotrol DiaBeta Amaryl
Meglitinides	Stimulates insulin, may cause weight gain, short acting	Repaglinide Nateglinide	Prandin Starlix
Biguanides	Improves insulin sensitivity, does not cause weight gain	Metformin	Glucophage
Thiazolidinediones	Decreases insulin resistance, causes water retention, can increase cholesterol	Pioglitazone	Actos
Alpha-glucosidase inhibitors	Delays intestinal absorption of carbohydrate, can cause nausea and diarrhea, does not cause weight gain)	Acarbose Miglitol	Precose Glyset
Dipeptidyl-peptidase-4 inhibitors	Decreases liver glucagon, slows down GLP-1 degradation, can cause headache, does not cause weight gain	Saxagliptin Sitagliptin	Onglyza Januvia

Source: University of Pittsburgh School of Health Science.

Of all the oral medications indicated in the previous table, metformin is used most often. When compared to the other oral diabetic medications, it is associated with increased longevity. This may be because it can help with weight management and the prevention of low blood sugar. Metformin is called an "insulin sensitizer" because it makes your own insulin work better.

The second-most common oral medication indicated in the table is glipizide. This stimulates the pancreas to produce a steady increase of insulin. When taking it, eat three meals and a snack a day to prevent low blood sugar.

 RED FLAG

If you are taking Actos and suddenly gain a lot of weight, experience shortness of breath, or experience swelling in your arms, hands, feet or ankles, tell your doctor. This medication can cause water retention, and can cause or worsen congestive heart failure in some people. Recent FDA notices have brought this to the public's attention.

Noninsulin Injections

The following table lists some noninsulin injection medications for diabetes that you might want to try if weight loss is one of your goals. These injections are also helpful because they encourage growth of insulin-secreting cells (islet cells in the pancreas) and can help you better control your blood sugar. Consult with your doctor about these.

Byetta and Victoza injections have a glucagon-like peptide receptor (GLP-1), which is a naturally occurring substance in the body that helps the pancreas release the right amount of insulin when blood sugar levels are high.

Symlin injections have a synthetic version of a hormone called amylin. Amylin is a naturally occurring substance in the body that helps make insulin work better. In nondiabetic individuals, glucose control depends not only on insulin but also on amylin. In diabetic people the ability to produce enough amylin is impaired.

Noninsulin Injections That Can Help with Weight Management

Generic Name	Brand Name (times taken/day)	Effects
Exenatide	Byetta (2x/day)	Helps with weight loss, slows down loss of GLP-1
Liraglutide	Victoza (1x/day)	
Pramlintide	Symlin (2–3x/day) (only used when taking insulin)	Mimetic incretin, helps with weight loss

Source: Fonseca, V. A., and K. D. Kulkarni. "Management of Type 2 Diabetes: Oral Agents, Insulin, and Injectables." J Am Diet Assoc. *2008; 108: S29-S33.*

Insulin

For a person without diabetes, insulin secretion and blood glucose levels simultaneously increase almost instantaneously when food is consumed. The insulin response is very precise and keeps the blood sugar in a healthy range instantaneously.

If you have diabetes, your insulin response must be managed. Type 1 diabetics will need to take insulin, and if you are a type 2 diabetic, you may also need to take insulin along with oral medications..

There are many types of insulin and it comes in different containers such as vials, syringes, reusable and disposable insulin pens, and insulin pumps. Some insulins can be mixed in order to provide combination effects, others cannot. Your doctor and diabetes educator will show you which ones you can mix and how to administer insulin.

As shown in the following table, the types of insulin are divided into four categories based on when they start working (onset), when they reach the highest level in your body (peak), and how long they stay in your body (duration). The categories include rapid-acting insulin, short-acting insulin, intermediate-acting insulin, and long-acting insulin. The type of insulin you will need to take depends on what your goals are and what type of insurance coverage you have.

Whatever type of insulin you choose, you will need to take that insulin at a time when it will do you the most good. This table will be useful to check the insulin your doctor has prescribed for you to understand how it works. You may use other forms of insulin at times if your needs change or if your doctor feels a different insulin would give you better blood glucose control.

Onset, Peak, and Duration Times of Different Types of Insulin

Insulin Types	Onset	Peak	Duration
Rapid:			
Humalog(lispro)	5–15 min.	30–90 min.	3–5 hrs.
Novolog (aspart)			
Apidra (glulisine)			
Short Acting:			
Humulin R (regular)	30 min.	2–4 hrs.	4–8 hrs.
Novolin R (regular)			
Intermediate Acting:			
Humulin N (NPH)	1½–4 hrs.	4–12 hrs.	10–24 hrs.
Novolin N (NPH)			
Combinations:			
Humalog Mix 75/25	15–30 min.	1–6½ hrs.	18–24 hrs.
Novolog Mix			
Humalog Mix 50/50			

continues

continued

Insulin Types	Onset	Peak	Duration
Long Acting:			
Lantus (glargine)	1–4 hrs.	Minimal	24 hrs.
Levemir (determir)			

Source: University of Pittsburgh School of Health Science.

Matching Blood Glucose Peaks

If you are taking insulin, it is important to match the peak time of your insulin to the peak time of your blood sugar levels. Typically your blood sugar will peak at an average of one hour after the start of a mixed meal (containing protein, carbohydrate, and fat). Knowing this can better help you identify the best time to take your insulin.

Insulin Peaks

When taking rapid-acting insulin like Humalog or Novolog, it is important to take it right before the meal. This is because after one hour of injecting rapid-acting insulin, your blood insulin will peak. As long as you match the peak glucose to the peak insulin times, you will get good results.

Weight Gain and Insulin

Taking insulin will often cause weight gain when you first start treatment; you had weight loss because your cells did not get glucose without insulin. Some weight gain may be warranted, but gaining excess weight can cause further insulin resistance and increase the likelihood of complications. If you are taking insulin and have been gaining weight, you can lose weight by changing your diet and by exercising, and/or by taking a noninsulin injection called Symlin (see the earlier table, "Noninsulin Injections That Can Help with Weight Management").

If you decrease the amount of carbohydrate food you eat or increase your activity level, you will need to slightly decrease the amount of insulin that you are taking in order to avoid a low blood sugar. Likewise, if you take Symlin, you also need to decrease the amount of insulin you're taking. In either case, make sure you frequently monitor your blood sugar.

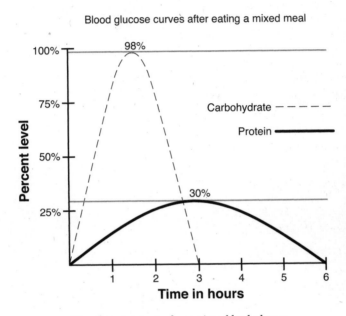

How fast nutrients change into blood glucose.

Hypoglycemia

When you use insulin or an insulin-stimulating oral medication such as glipizide (Glucotrol), it is important to be prepared to avoid a *hypoglycemic* episode. These medications are very effective in lowering your blood sugar. If you forget to eat on time, or happen to exercise too much and still take your usual amount of insulin, your blood sugar can go too low. Balance is the key. You will learn how to best avoid hypoglycemia by monitoring your blood sugar and following the directions of your doctor or diabetes educator.

DEFINITION

Hypoglycemia is a abnormally low blood sugar that can cause impairment of brain function. There are mild to serious degrees of hypoglycemia, causing problems from irritability and shakiness to a severe situation resulting in losing consciousness or having a seizure.

Early symptoms of a low blood glucose level include:

- Sweating
- Dizziness
- Fainting
- Slurred speech
- Tremors
- Headache
- Restlessness
- Irritability
- Weakness
- Poor concentration

Many people who have low blood glucose levels are not aware of it. Consequently, it is important to check blood glucose levels on a scheduled basis or if any of the previous symptoms are present.

Treatment

In the event of low blood glucose, it is important to have a hypoglycemic plan to follow. The American Diabetes Association (ADA) advises using the following guidelines in treating hypoglycemia.

1. If the blood glucose is <70 mg/dL on your meter, give 15 to 20 grams of a carbohydrate. Examples of 15 grams of carbohydrate include the following:

    - ½ cup regular soda
    - 3 glucose tablets
    - 1 tube Glutose 15
    - 3 sugar cubes or 3 packets sugar
    - 5 Lifesaver candies

2. Wait 15 minutes, then recheck blood glucose. If it's still <70 mg/dL, repeat step 1.

3. After blood glucose is >70, follow up with a more substantial snack or meal containing carbohydrates, proteins, and fat, if the next meal is more than 2 hours away.

Preferred carbohydrate sources to use for hypoglycemia include glucose, dextrose, or sucrose. Dextrose and glucose are simple sugars that are absorbed very quickly, and sucrose (table sugar) contains glucose and can also be absorbed quickly. Fruit juices and fruits take a longer time to raise blood sugar levels because fructose must be converted to glucose in the liver before entering blood circulation. Drinks with high-fructose corn syrup are also not recommended. Sources of glucose, dextrose, or sucrose include regular soda, glucose tablets, Glutose tubes, sugar cubes or packets of sugar, and Lifesaver candies.

Continuous Glucose Monitoring

If hypoglycemia is a frequent problem and you're already checking your blood sugar frequently, you can try a continuous glucose monitoring (CGM) device, which is attached just under the skin in the abdomen. The device can read blood glucose levels every few minutes and give a paper or computer graph of almost real-time glucose usage. Except for the copay, CGM devices are generally covered by most major insurance companies.

The CGM device is not a replacement for standard blood sugar monitoring. It is used only to find trends in your blood sugar and its placement only tests for 72 hours. The information derived from the monitor can help determine your treatment plan.

Medication Interactions

Drug interactions with your diabetic medication are common. Be sure to tell your pharmacist about all the medications, vitamins, and herbal supplements you are currently taking and to inquire about any possible interactions. Drugs are mostly eliminated by the liver and kidneys. If you overload your system with too many medications at one time, serious consequences can arise. You and your diabetes care team want to see that you protect yourself by taking medications correctly.

 RED FLAG

Several medications (such as prednisone, tacrolimus, phenytoin, atenolol, and carvediol) can increase your blood sugar. When taking these medications, you may need to adjust your diabetic medications to maintain good blood sugar control. Be sure to ask your doctor how to do this.

Several diabetic medications can also increase the need for some vitamins and minerals. Most diabetic people have better blood glucose levels when taking a B-complex vitamin and a magnesium supplement. See Chapter 9 for more details.

Planning Your Care

When determining how best to manage your medications, be prepared for all situations. Here's a checklist:

- Use a glucose meter to monitor your blood sugar on a regular basis. Take the meter with you when you leave your house, or purchase a second meter to have at work. Don't leave it in a hot or very cold car, but keep at room temperature.

- Determine your health goals. If you want to lose weight, ask your doctor about medications that won't make you gain weight. (See Chapters 6, 7, and 8 on weight management, behavior changing, and exercise.)

- Coordinate your medication with your diet and exercise. Pay attention to when your insulin peaks and how long it stays in your body.

- Be sure to carry a form of glucose or sucrose (Lifesaver candies, glucose tablets, sugar packets, etc.) if you are taking insulin or an oral diabetic medication that increases insulin production.

- When you are traveling, medication, insulin, and test strips need to be stored in a cool environment. They can be damaged by heat in just a couple of minutes.

- At home, store medications according to how your pharmacist or diabetes educator tells you.

- If you are going out all day, take along your insulin, your medications, some water, and some food in an insulated cooler.

Eating to Control Blood Sugar

After a long day at work, James couldn't wait to get home. He was ravenous, and he hoped that his wife, Julie, had cooked his favorite dinner of steak, biscuits, and mashed potatoes with gravy. As he entered the house he smelled mint leaves and vinegar. He walked up to Julie and asked, "Honey, what's for dinner?"

Julie looked directly at James and said, "How does salmon, a vegetable salad, and a small baked potato sound to you?"

James was taken aback. "Really, fish? We haven't had that for a while … and why the 'small' potato?" Julie stepped over to the kitchen counter and picked up an envelope. That's when James remembered that he had told Julie that she could look at the lab results his doctor had given him. His doctor had told him that he was prediabetic and that he had to cut down on his carbohydrates. His only thought had been, "What's a carbohydrate?"

It's not about the fish or steak. It's about the potatoes and biscuits, and James will be happy to know he can still have some of his favorite foods in moderate amounts. This chapter discusses basic food nutrient components, and explains how each of these affects blood sugar levels. It also details planning methods for good blood glucose control.

Three Basic Nutrients in Food

The three basic nutrient components in food that contribute to calorie consumption are protein, fat, and carbohydrates. Of the three, carbohydrates have the biggest impact on your blood sugar.

Protein

Foods that are mostly protein include meat, poultry, fish, eggs, and hard cheese. About 40 percent of these foods break down (metabolize) into blood sugar. This does not happen very quickly. By the time protein is finally turned into blood sugar, about two-and-a-half to three hours have elapsed; this is why protein does not have as big an impact on blood sugar levels as carbohydrates.

Fat

Foods high in fat include oil, butter, mayonnaise, avocadoes, nuts, and seeds. By themselves, fats hardly affect the blood sugar. However, since fat makes up more than 35 percent of the calories in a meal and is often eaten with a lot of carbohydrate foods at one time, there is a delayed blood sugar response. This is because high amounts of fat can slow down the absorption of a meal. In addition, there is evidence that eating a higher fat diet on a regular basis can cause insulin resistance.

Carbohydrates

Carbohydrates have a huge impact on blood sugar. About 98 percent of these foods are metabolized into blood glucose. Foods like potatoes, rice, pasta, bread, fruit, fruit juice, milk, desserts, table sugar, honey, agave, and syrup are all high in carbohydrates.

Carbohydrate food contains "hidden" sugars. When they are consumed, the "hidden" sugar metabolizes into blood sugar. Here are some hidden sugars in carbohydrate foods:

- Starches (for example, rice, potatoes, bread): *polysaccharides*
- Fruit: fructose, mannose, and glucose
- Milk: lactose and galactose
- Table sugar (sucrose): glucose and fructose

> **DEFINITION**
>
> **Polysaccharide** is defined as many sugars occurring together. Some of the common sugars a polysaccharide contains include glucose, mannose, and galactose.

It's All About Carbohydrates

Diabetics are told to watch their carbohydrates, and people who want to lose weight are told to limit or avoid carbohydrates. Popular plans such as the Atkin's, South Beach, and Zone diets are designed to lower the total carbohydrate intake. Do people with diabetes need to totally avoid carbohydrates? Can you lose weight on a low carbohydrate diet even if you eat more calories than you need? How fast do carbohydrates turn into sugar? If some carbohydrates are allowed, how much is too much? All of these questions are about to be answered.

How Fast?

Just because you have diabetes does not mean that you need to totally avoid carbohydrates. They are not bad; in fact, they give us energy to keep our muscles and heart running smoothly and help our brain function. You do need to monitor your carbohydrate intake, however.

How fast do carbohydrates turn into blood sugar? The answer is quickly! About one hour after eating a carbohydrate, your blood sugar level will be at its highest point. When this happens, the body needs insulin to help lower your blood sugar. For a person without diabetes, insulin secretion and blood sugar levels simultaneously increase when food is consumed. However, for someone with type 2 diabetes and prediabetes, insulin secretions and insulin sensitivity are compromised. Consequently, this means that not as much carbohydrate food is tolerated at one time. In addition, some people with diabetes may need medication to increase their ability to tolerate carbohydrates.

How Much?

Carbohydrates should be eaten in smaller amounts and be evenly distributed throughout the day. Three small meals and two snacks, spread out about three to four hours apart during a day, is a much better eating plan than two large meals a day.

The actual amount of carbohydrates best tolerated in one meal will be different from person to person. Some people will be fine if they consume 60 grams of carbohydrates in a meal, but others may only be able to consume 30 grams of carbohydrates in a meal. The amount of tolerance depends on many factors, including your activity level, degree of insulin resistance, medications taken, and rate of metabolism.

An easy way to find out how many carbohydrate grams you can tolerate is to check your blood sugar level two hours after eating a specified amount of carbohydrates. Two hours after your meal, your blood sugar should be <180 and preferably ≤140. It is important to know your tolerance level of carbohydrate foods because each episode of high blood sugar can result in the production of free radicals, leading to damage in your blood vessels.

Planning Methods

Meal planning approaches that can be used to estimate carbohydrate intake include carbohydrate counting, the American Diabetes Association (ADA) exchange system, plate methods, food guide pyramid methods, and the glycemic index (GI). Some of these approaches are more accurate than others in determining amounts of carbohydrate intake.

Carbohydrate Counting

With carbohydrate counting, carbohydrate foods (such as starchy vegetables, grains, fruits, milk, and foods with added sugars) are weighed or measured at a meal. Total carbohydrate *grams* in the food are then added up. Generally, a carbohydrate counter device or book is used as a reference when determining amounts of carbohydrate grams. Carbohydrate counters can be found online, in bookstores, and in many merchandise stores. Carbohydrate counting is the most accurate method of determining actual carbohydrate grams eaten and should be used in the following situations:

- When you want more precise control of your blood sugar
- When using a specified amount of insulin for a specified amount of carbohydrate grams
- When your blood sugar is not well controlled using other methods of meal planning

DEFINITION

A **gram** is a measurement that is often used to measure food nutrients such as protein, fat, and carbohydrates. Comparatively, 28 grams equals about 1 ounce.

The number of carbohydrate grams varies according to the amount of water and fiber present in the food. The more water or fiber a food contains, the smaller the carbohydrate content. Examples of equal grams of carbohydrates in foods with varying degrees of water content are as follows:

- 1 tablespoon granulated sugar = 15 grams
- 2 tablespoons raisins = 15 grams
- ½ cup applesauce = 15 grams
- 1 cup cantaloupe = 15 grams

The following table shows the carbohydrate content of a typical dinner.

Example Meal Plan Using Carbohydrate Counting

Food	Amount	Carbohydrate Grams
Roasted chicken	3 oz.	0
Tossed salad (lettuce, cucumbers, radishes, green peppers)	2 cups	5
Oil and vinegar	2 TB.	0
Baked yam	8 oz.	30
Sugar-free, fat-free ice cream	½ cup	15

Total Meal Carbohydrates: 50 grams

Common carbohydrate amounts at a meal are between 45 and 75 grams. Each meal can be planned ahead of time in order to make it easier to keep carbohydrate amounts more accurate. This might sound like a lot of work at first; however, once you get a pattern started, it becomes second nature.

Your doctor will instruct you to use a specific amount of insulin for a specific amount of carbohydrate. Check your blood sugar prior to the meal and two hours after the meal in order to see if the amount of insulin you used for the amount of carbohydrate grams you ate is appropriate. If your blood sugar is off, you may need to adjust your insulin or food intake. Talk to your diabetes educator or endocrinologist before making any insulin changes.

American Diabetic Exchange System

The ADA has developed a system to estimate carbohydrate amounts. It is not as accurate as carbohydrate counting, but it is more accurate than using the plate and pyramid methods to estimate carbohydrate amounts. You'll learn more about the plate method later in this chapter, and find out about the pyramid method in Chapter 5.

Major Food Exchange Groups

With the ADA exchange system, foods are grouped into three major categories: carbohydrates, protein, and fats:

- The carbohydrate category includes starchy foods, fruit, milk, milk products, and sugar-containing foods. The nonstarchy vegetables like broccoli and asparagus are also carbohydrate, but have lower carbohydrate content than the other carbohydrate foods. Starchy foods such as dried beans, potatoes, and corn contain more carbohydrates.
- The protein category includes four sections: lean meat/substitutes, moderate fat meats, high-fat meats, and plant-based proteins.
- The fat category includes three sections: monounsaturated fats, polyunsaturated fats, and saturated fats (see Chapter 6).

All food measurements listed in each major category are listed in quantities that contain about equal amounts of either carbohydrate grams, protein grams, or fat grams. Just like exchanging equal amounts of money (four quarters for one dollar), the foods listed in each category work in a similar way. Each food quantity listed within a specific category is exchangeable to another food within that same category because they have equal amounts of the specified basic food nutrient.

Carbohydrate Exchange

The most important part of the exchange system is the carbohydrate exchange. A carbohydrate exchange is 15 grams (g) of carbohydrate. Here is an example of how it works:

> 1 small apple (15 g) = $\frac{1}{2}$ cup corn (15 g) = $\frac{1}{3}$ cup pasta (15 g) = 1 cup plain yogurt (15 g)

Example carbohydrate foods with their serving sizes for each carbohydrate category are listed in the following table. Each of these servings represents one carbohydrate exchange. The type of food example shown in the table can come in various forms and still have about the same amount of carbohydrates. For example, one slice of bread or $\frac{1}{3}$ cup of rice, whether it is whole grain or white, will still contain 15 grams of carbohydrates. In addition, skim milk or whole milk, even though the fat content is different, contains about the same amount of carbohydrate grams.

Food shown in the exchange list form are averages of carbohydrate grams. To get more specific you will need to read labels or check a more detailed carbohydrate counter source.

Food Lists for Major Carbohydrate Groups*

Starches	Fruit	Milk	Sweets
1 slice bread	1 small fruit	1 cup milk	1-inch square cake, unfrosted
1 tortilla (6 in.)	$\frac{1}{2}$ cup canned fruit	1 cup plain yogurt	2 small cookies
$\frac{1}{2}$ cup cooked cereal	$\frac{1}{4}$ cup dried fruit	1 cup soy milk	$\frac{1}{2}$ cup ice cream

Starches	Fruit	Milk	Sweets
¾ cup ready-to-eat cereal	½ cup juice		¼ cup sherbet
⅓ cup cooked pasta or rice	1 cup melon or berries		1 TB. jam, honey, or sugar
3 cups popcorn	2 TB. raisins		2 TB. light syrup

One serving = approximately 15 g carbohydrates
Source: American Dietetic Association.

See an example of the ADA exchange lists in the following table. This example shows how many carbohydrate, protein, and fat grams as well as how many calories are in each of the food groups.

ADA Food Exchange System

Food Sections	Carbohydrate Grams	Protein/ Meat Grams	Fat Grams	Calories
Starch	15	3	0	80
Fruit	15	0	0	60
Milk, fat free	12	8	0	90
Milk, low fat	12	8	5	120
Milk, whole	12	8	8	150
Vegetables, nonstarch	5	2	0	25
Meat/lean	0	7	0–3	35
Meat/medium fat	0	7	4–7	55
Meat/high fat	0	7	8+	100
Plant-based proteins	Varies	7	Varies	Varies
Fats	0	0	5	45

Source: American Dietetic Association.

✎ **TO YOUR HEALTH**

To purchase an ADA Exchange booklet, go online to eatright.org.

Determining Carbohydrates, Fat, and Protein Exchanges and Calories

In addition to counting carbohydrates by the exchange method, you may want to determine specific calorie amounts, especially if you are interested in weight control. Just because an individual eats a low-carbohydrate diet does not mean he will lose weight. He needs to also decrease his total calorie intake. For help with how many calories you need for weight management, see Chapter 6.

When using the ADA system for menu planning, you take the total number of calories you want to take in and multiply it by the percentage of carbohydrate, protein, and fat you want. For example, if you want a 1,600-calorie meal plan and 55 percent of the calories from carbohydrates, 20 percent from protein, and 25 percent from fat, multiply 1,600 calories by .55 for carbohydrate calories, by .20 for protein calories, and by .25 for fat calories.

To find total carbohydrate grams, divide the total carbohydrate calories by 4. There are 4 calories in each gram of carbohydrate. To find total protein grams, divide the total protein calories by 4. Protein also has 4 calories per gram. To find total fat grams, divide the total fat calories by 9. There are 9 calories in 1 gram of fat.

Example: Determining percent of protein, carbohydrate, and fat grams for a 1,600-calorie diet

Total calories: 1,600

55% for carbohydrate: $1,600 \times .55 = 880$ calories $\div 4 = 220$ g

20% for protein: $1,600 \times .20 = 320$ calories $\div 4 = 80$ g protein

25% for fat: $1,600 \times .25 = 400$ calories $\div 9 = 44.4$ g fat

With the total protein, carbohydrate, and fat gram information, you can find how many exchanges you need by doing a little more math. To determine carbohydrate exchanges, take the total carbohydrate grams and divide by 15. This is because there are 15 grams of carbohydrates in each carbohydrate exchange. For example, using the 1,600-calorie diet that is 55 percent carbohydrates and has 220 carbohydrate grams, divide 15 to get total carbohydrate exchanges.

Example: Determining the number of carbohydrate exchanges to use

Total carbohydrate grams = 220 grams

> 220 grams/15 grams = 14.66 or about 15 carbohydrate exchanges

These carbohydrate exchanges are divided into meals and snacks. Remember the carbohydrate exchanges can be a starch, fruit, or milk. In the following table, all carbohydrate exchanges are shown in bold.

ADA Meal 15 Carbohydrate Exchanges for the Day

Breakfast	Lunch	Dinner	Afternoon Snack	Evening Snack
1 lean meat	2 lean meat	3 lean meat		
1 low-fat milk	**1 low-fat milk**			
0–1 vegetable	2 vegetable	2 vegetable		
2 starch	**2 starch**	**2 starch**		**2 starch**
1 fruit		**1 fruit**	**2 fruit**	**1 fruit**
2 fat	2 fat	2 fat	2 fat	

In this meal plan there are three carbohydrate exchanges (45 g carbohydrates) used per meal. Depending on what you can tolerate, the amount of carbohydrate exchanges or total carbohydrate grams per meal and snack time can be adjusted. Some diabetic middle-age and sedentary individuals find that they can only consume about 45 grams of carbohydrates per eating session before they will compromise their blood glucose control. Other diabetic people may have good blood glucose control with more carbohydrates, and some may need even less than 45 grams per meal or snack.

Remember to check how many carbohydrate grams are tolerated, as indicated earlier, it can be helpful to test the blood glucose levels two hours after eating.

To see more examples of exchange portions for nonstarchy vegetables, starches, protein, and fat, see the Exchange Lists for Diabetics (American Dietetic Association, American Diabetes Association, 2008).

Plate Methods

Carbohydrate counting and using the ADA exchange system can be overwhelming for some of us. Luckily, there are some visual planning methods that may work better for you, although they are not quite as accurate as carbohydrate counting or using the ADA exchange system.

Diabetic Plate Method

A common and easy-to-follow visual planner is a diabetic plate method. One half of the plate is labeled nonstarchy vegetables, one fourth labeled protein, and one fourth labeled starchy foods. The fruit and milk groups are optional and are shown as icons outside the plate. The approximate total carbohydrate count for this if the milk or fruit options were used is about 45 to 60 grams.

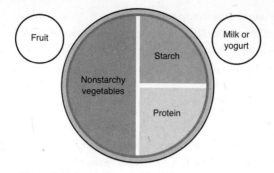

Typical diabetic plate method for meal planning.

MyPlate Method

A plate method introduced in June 2011 by the United States
Department of Agriculture (USDA) and U.S. Department
of Health and Human Services (HHS) is called the MyPlate
method. MyPlate was created as an initiative of the new 2010
Dietary Guidelines. It replaced the USDA MyPyramid method
to help engage more Americans to follow a healthy diet. The
MyPlate guideline has four pie-shaped plate divisions, where
approximately one fourth is from protein, one fourth from
grains, one fourth from fruit, and one fourth from vegetables.
A dairy group serving is also part of the meal and is shown as a
circle to the side of the plate. The message of the MyPlate image
is to eat meals that include the five food categories (vegetables,
fruit, protein, grains, and dairy) in the proportions shown.

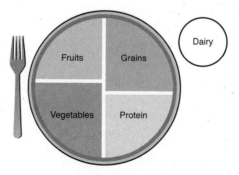

MyPlate method for meal planning.

The MyPlate website (choosemyplate.gov) provides the basic guidelines from the 2010 Dietary Guidelines for Americans (DGA), which advocates portion control; eating slowly and more mindfully; using smaller plates; and eating more vegetables, fruits, whole grains, and fat-free or 1-percent-fat milk products.

The differences between MyPlate method and the diabetic plate method is the amount of total carbohydrate grams on the left side of each plate. The diabetic plate has one half of the plate designated for nonstarchy (lower carbohydrate) vegetables, whereas MyPlate has one fourth of the plate designated for fruit and one fourth for vegetables. Since fruit is higher carbohydrate content than nonstarchy veggies and the type of vegetable is not defined on the MyPlate method, the total amount of carbohydrate foods from using this method will be higher.

If you use MyPlate method, you can change the fruit section with nonstarchy vegetables, resulting in one half of your plate filled with nonstarchy vegetables. Examples of higher carbohydrate vegetables include corn, peas, and winter squash. Examples of nonstarchy vegetables include broccoli, summer squash, and green beans.

 RED FLAG

Do not pile high mounds of food on any part of your plate, whether using a typical diabetic plate plan or the MyPlate version. If you do, the carbohydrate amounts will be significantly higher.

GI Diabetic Plate Method

I developed the glycemic index (GI) diabetic plate method, in which 50 percent of the plate is designated for nonstarchy vegetables, 25 percent for carbohydrate foods, 20 percent for lean protein, and about 5 percent for healthy fats. If using this plate method, the total carbohydrate grams for the meal will be lower than it is with the typical diabetic or MyPlate plate methods.

Approximate total carbohydrate intake for the GI plate method is 15 to 30 grams. This can be for you if you want to cut back on total carbohydrate intake consumed at one time, but don't want to count carbohydrates or use the ADA exchange system.

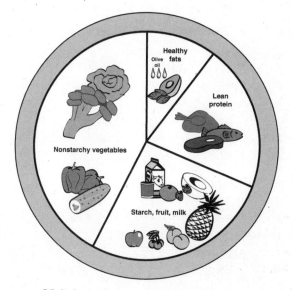

GI diabetic plate method for meal planning.

Determining the Best Method for You

Are you a more detailed person who likes precision? Do you want to use a specific amount of insulin for a specific amount of carbohydrate grams? If your answer is yes to either of these questions, then the carbohydrate counting method or the ADA exchange system method of monitoring can work well for you.

If you do better with less detail, or find it too hard or cumbersome to count carbohydrates, then using a format such as the plate method for monitoring carbohydrate intake might be best for you.

Using the Glycemic Index

Rita, a newly diagnosed diabetic, just learned how to use the glycemic index with carbohydrate counting. Excited to try some new low GI recipes, she called her friend Angela and asked, "Angela, can you come over to eat on Friday? I'm so excited; I'm going to make a GI dinner!"

Angela, who is pretty, single, and interested in meeting men, held the phone closer to her ear before speaking. "You're fixing dinner for a soldier? I've never dated a soldier before. That is exciting! What shall I wear?"

Angela is about to find out exactly what Rita had in mind. Perhaps she won't be too disappointed when she finds out that eating a low GI meal can be both delicious and satisfying. Simultaneously, Rita may find that using foods with a lower GI can help decrease appetite and control blood glucose levels. This chapter will show you how to use the glycemic index in conjunction with carbohydrate planning.

Defining and Ranking the GI

The most important factor when controlling blood sugar is the amount of carbohydrates consumed, but the type of carbohydrates also plays an important role. Even if you keep your carbohydrate grams equal from meal to meal, you will find that some carbohydrates change into blood sugar to a greater degree than others. How much the *glycemic index (GI)* will affect your blood sugar may be somewhat different from person to person, but in general, carbohydrates with lower GI foods will help keep your blood sugar lower and more stable than carbohydrates with a higher GI. Foods that contain mostly fats (such as oils and butter) or primarily protein (such as meat and chicken) are not considered to be significant when measuring GI because they do not have a big impact on our blood sugar. Carbohydrates, however, have a big impact. About 98 percent of carbohydrates turn into blood sugar.

> **DEFINITION**
>
> The **glycemic index (GI)** measures the effects that a carbohydrate food has on blood glucose levels.

Is Using the GI Effective?

Using the GI method in choosing carbohydrate foods has been shown to be effective in keeping blood glucose levels lower and more stable. The GI term was made popular in the early 1980s with the work of Dr. David J. Jenkins and Dr. Thomas Wolever at the University of Toronto, and with Dr. Jennie Brand-Miller, RD, at the University of Sydney. Their research was conducted to determine which foods are most helpful for people with diabetes. Their work included observation and measurement of blood glucose levels in test subjects who ate the same amount of carbohydrate, but from different sources. A standard portion of food that contained 50 grams of carbohydrates was given to each individual to eat. After eating, each person's blood sugar was tested every 10 minutes for one hour, then every 15 minutes for the second hour, and every 30 minutes for the third hour.

In these observations, blood glucose differences were recorded as related to the foods being tested. All of the foods tested were assigned a number based on the blood glucose response measured on each test subject. Oral glucose (the form of blood sugar) was used as the standard reference number, and was given a rank of 100. All the other foods were ranked on a scale from 0 to 100.

GI Ranking

Foods assigned a lower number (lower GI) are better for you. They can help prevent blood sugar spikes and keep your blood sugar more stable. Foods assigned a higher number (higher GI) are not so good for you. They can raise your blood sugar faster and to a greater degree. GI numbers are ranked in categories of low, moderate, and high, as indicated in the following table.

GI Number Ranks

Numbers	GI Rank
70–100	High
55–70	Moderate
55 or lower	Low

Source: The Glucose Revolution, The Authoritative Guide to the Glycemic Index, *Jennie Brand-Miller et.al. New York: Marlowe & Company; July 1999.*

GI Variations

The GI of any one food can vary depending on several factors. This is often due to the differences in the molecular structure of starches and sugars that occur naturally in food.

Cooking

The GI of food not only changes because of natural differences in the molecular structure of starches and sugars, but also because of the way the food was processed. Starches in foods like pasta, breads, and muffins absorb water during the cooking process and then swell and rupture in a process called gelatinization. When this happens, the food becomes easier for the body to break down into blood sugar. The easier it is to break down food into blood sugar, the bigger the impact there will be on elevating blood glucose levels. In addition, the longer the food is cooked, the worse it is for your blood sugar. Well-cooked foods have a higher GI than less cooked foods. For example, starches such as rice or pasta cooked for 30 minutes have a higher GI than if cooked for 15 minutes.

In addition, vegetables such as carrots or beets eaten raw have a lower GI than if they were cooked, and just like with rice and pasta, the longer these vegetables are cooked, the higher their GI will be.

TO YOUR HEALTH

To obtain a lower GI, use al dente cooking for pasta, vegetables, and rice. Al dente cooking is cooked tender, but firm to the bite. It takes approximately 8 minutes to cook elbow-shaped pasta to an al dente texture.

Shape and Density

In general, pasta has a lower GI value than many other starches. This is due to its shape and density, which when cooking causes some physical entrapment of uncooked (ungelatinized) starch granules within its structure. Other examples of more dense starches include tortillas and flat breads. All of these products tend to have a lower GI.

Molecular Structure of Starch

The type of starch you eat can make a difference when it comes to your blood sugar. Some starches have a lower GI and some can be high.

Pure starch is a white, tasteless, and odorless powder that does not dissolve in cold water or alcohol. It consists of two types of molecules: the linear long-chained straight (amylose) molecule, and the branched short-chained (amylopectin) molecule. A starch containing a lot of amylose has a lower GI. A starch containing a lot of amylopectin has a higher GI. This is because the branched short-chain molecule has more exposed area for the body's digestive enzymes (secreted in the stomach and intestine) to work on than the long-chain straight starch molecule.

Some foods naturally have more amylopectin and some more amylose. Foods high in amylose (low glycemic) include unripe bananas, legumes, peas, and intact whole grains. Foods high in amylopectin (high glycemic) include baked potatoes, white rice, and refined grains.

Changing Amylopectin into Amylose

Even though a baked potato has a high amount of amylopectin starch (high glycemic), if you eat it hot from the oven, the GI can change if it is put into the refrigerator. This is because cooling a starchy food changes the way the molecules line up. Once cooled, some of the structure can change from amylopectin starch into amylose starch, thereby lowering the GI. If you reheat the once cooked and cooled potato, it will change the GI upward again, but not as high as it was when initially baked (then fluffy in texture). Some of the changed starch structure by cooling the potato stays even if cooked again.

Starches can also be chemically modified in order to obtain a lower GI. Manufactured starch like this is often referred to as *resistant starch*. Examples of resistant starches on the market include products such as Hi-maize corn and ActiStar starch.

> **DEFINITION**
>
> **Resistant starch** is a carbohydrate that is high in amylose molecules and resists breakdown and absorption in the small intestine. It is often considered a type of dietary fiber because much of it passes through the small intestine unabsorbed to the large intestine, where it acts like fiber.

To help lower and/or slow down the carbohydrate absorption, resistant starches have been added to many products in the supermarket, such as ExtendBar, Aunt Millie's Whole-Grain Muffins, and Ener-G Foods Wylde Pretzels. However, if you use these products you will still need to read the food labels and count carbohydrate grams. Some of these products are higher in fiber, so you will end up consuming less overall carbohydrate grams. For foods that have 5 grams of fiber or more per serving, the American Diabetic Association recommends subtracting one half of the total fiber content from total carbohydrate grams.

To determine how each product affects you, it is wise to monitor your blood sugar two hours after the meal. Depending on if you want strict or moderate glucose control, your two-hour blood glucose goal should be between 140mg/dl and 180mg/dl.

Processing

Processing can change the GI of a food. Processing fruit into fruit juice or vegetables into vegetable juice removes fiber and changes a food's structure. Consequently, the GI increases. Structure changes can also occur with various types of mixing and grinding methods. For example, mashed potatoes have a higher GI than a whole potato, and stone-ground intact wheat bread has a lower GI than blended wheat bread. The more a food is processed into smaller particles, the higher the GI.

Other Effects

Different variety of grains, fruits, or vegetables can also have different GIs. For example, basmati brown rice has a lower GI than most short-grain brown rice, and red potatoes have a lower GI than white potatoes.

Adding fat or protein to carbohydrates can decrease the GI. Mashed potatoes by themselves have a higher GI than mashed potatoes with gravy and chicken.

Maturation of vegetables and fruit can also change the GI. The riper fruit or vegetable is, the higher GI. For example, unripe bananas have a lower GI than ripe ones.

Both soluble and insoluble fiber will help decrease the GI value. Insoluble fiber, which is hard like wheat bran and celery stalks, can act as a physical barrier that prevents enzymes from attacking the food. Soluble fiber, which is viscous and sticky like pectin and guar gum, lowers the GI by slowing down the speed of food transit time in the intestine.

Finally, even the pH of a food can make a difference. Making the food more acidic by adding vinegar creates a lower pH and can make the GI of the entire meal lower. According to one study, the more vinegar used in a meal, the bigger the impact it had on lowering the GI and ultimately the blood sugar. The type of vinegar used was apple cider. Be careful, though: using more than two tablespoons of apple cider vinegar at one meal caused mouth, throat, and stomach irritation for some people in the study.

GI with the Use of Medication and Insulin

When lower glycemic foods are eaten, you will find that your blood sugar peak may occur slightly later and to a lesser degree than when eating higher glycemic foods. Knowing this may enable you to adjust your insulin downward slightly. The key, though, is to determine the effect lower GI meals have on you and to let your doctor know before making a medication change. To find out the effect, monitor your blood sugar level two hours after eating. Bring in your blood sugar monitoring log with you when visiting your diabetes provider or doctor to help them determine the direction you need to take with your medication or diet.

Glycemic Load (GL)

Because both GI and the amount of carbohydrate have an impact on your blood sugar, you may want to use a method of monitoring that does both. A formula that measures both is called the *glycemic load (GL)*.

📖 **DEFINITION**

The **glycemic load (GL)** is a formula that measures the product of the glycemic index of a carbohydrate food and the amount of carbohydrate grams eaten.

The GL is found by first determining total carbohydrate grams, and then multiplying this number by its GI value divided by 100:

$$GL = (\text{number of carbohydrates} \times GI) \div 100 = \underline{\quad}$$

For example:

One large 4 oz. peach with 15 g carbohydrate and a GI of 42: GL = 15 × 42 = 630 ÷ 100 = 6.32

One small 3 oz. potato with 15 g carbohydrate and a GI of 92: GL = 15 × 92 = 1,380 ÷ 100 = 13.8

These examples show that the 3 oz. potato raises the blood-glucose level higher than one 4 oz. peach, even though the carbohydrate amount is the same. For a lower blood sugar effect, the peach is a better choice than the potato.

Using GL numbers to find good blood sugar control may work well for you if you are a detail-oriented person. You will need to have a GI foods list, a carbohydrate counter, and a calculator. For a GI food list and calculator you can visit the University of Sydney website: glycemicindex.com/foodSearch.php. For some GI book resources, see the Appendix. You may do these calculations of foods you commonly eat and keep your own table for quick reference. After you gain experience, these will be very simple calculations for a few new foods you add over time.

If you find doing the GL calculations a bit cumbersome, you may find that using a food pyramid or plate guide that emphasizes using a lower glycemic index, higher fiber, and unprocessed carbohydrates may work better for you. For the lower GI plate method, see Chapter 4.

Glycemic Index Food Pyramid

With guidance from Dr. Dana Clarke at the Utah Diabetes Center at the University of Utah Hospitals and Clinics, I developed a GI food pyramid for people with type 2 diabetes. This pyramid can help you combine both the GI and carbohydrate portion control.

The overall message of the pyramid: as you eat more foods from the lower part of the pyramid, your blood sugar will be lower, but as you eat more foods from the higher levels of the pyramid, your blood sugar will be higher.

Within the pyramid are serving guidelines for keeping the diet lower in overall carbohydrate and adequate in healthy fats, protein, and other needed nutrients.

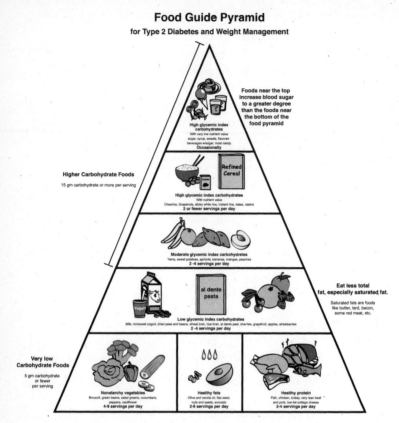

Diabetes and weight management food guide pyramid.

Five Levels of the Pyramid

This pyramid has five levels:

- At the bottom of the pyramid there are low GI, high fiber, and high nutrient-dense foods with very low or no carbohydrate content.

- The second tier of the pyramid has low GI, high fiber, and high nutrient-dense foods with moderate carbohydrate content.

- The third tier of the pyramid has moderate GI, high fiber, and moderately nutrient-dense foods with higher carbohydrate content.
- The fourth tier has high GI, little fiber, processed and less nutrient-dense foods that are high in carbohydrates.
- At the top of the pyramid there are carbohydrates that are highly refined, high glycemic, with no fiber, and no nutrient content.

Recommendations for Diabetic Glycemic Index Pyramid

To keep your blood sugar lower, it is recommended that you eat mostly foods from the bottom of the pyramid. Individual serving suggestions for all levels follow.

Bottom-tier, nonstarchy vegetables:

Servings: 4–9

Serving size: 1 cup raw or ½ cup cooked

Carbohydrates grams/serving: 5

Calories/serving: 25

Bottom-tier, lean protein foods:

Servings: 2–4

Serving size: 3 ounces fish, chicken, very lean beef, ½ cup low-fat cottage cheese

Carbohydrate grams/serving: 0–5

Calories/serving: 90–135

Bottom tier, healthy fats:

Servings: 2–6

Serving size: 1 teaspoon olive or canola oil, 2 tablespoons unsalted nuts and seeds

Carbohydrate grams/serving: 0–5

Calories/serving: 45

Second tier, low GI carbohydrates:

Servings: 2–4

Serving size: $\frac{1}{2}$ cup for cooked oats or fruit

Carbohydrate grams/serving: 15

Calories/serving: 60–90

Third tier, moderate GI carbohydrates:

Servings: 2–4

Serving size: $\frac{1}{2}$ cup cooked pasta or fruit

Carbohydrate grams/serving: 15

Calories/serving: 60–90

Fourth tier, high GI carbohydrates with nutrients:

Servings: 2 or fewer

Serving size: $\frac{1}{2}$ cup cooked cereal or 1 cup dry unsweetened cereal

Carbohydrate grams/serving: 15–45

Calories/serving: 80–135

Top of the pyramid, high GI, no nutrients:

Servings: occasional

Serving size: 1 cup soft drink, 1–2 ounces candy

Carbohydrate grams/serving: varies

Calories/serving: varies

Weight Management and Diabetes

Nicole had to look twice before she recognized her friend Bonnie at the class reunion. She hadn't seen Bonnie for five years, and at that time, Bonnie had just found out she had type 2 diabetes. Nicole thought, Wow, Bonnie must have lost about 30 pounds. No wonder I didn't recognize her!

Nicole walked over to Bonnie and smiled. "Bonnie, it's so good to see you. You look wonderful! Did you lose some weight?"

Bonnie's eyes lit up as she hugged her friend. "Nicole! I'm so happy to see you! Yes, I did lose some weight, and I feel so much better. Do you remember five years ago I was sick all the time and had to start taking diabetic medications? Well, now I no longer need the medications and I'm doing really well with controlling my blood sugar."

"Oh, Bonnie, I'm so glad for you. Please tell me how you lost your weight. I'd love to lose a little weight, too." Bonnie told Nicole how modifying her diet, using food journaling, exercising, and changing one of her medications had helped her lose weight.

Weight loss can become complex and overwhelming at times, but with a little focus and direction you too can achieve your goals. This chapter shows you how.

A Healthy Body Weight

Being at your right body weight can help prevent, improve, and sometimes even cure your diabetes. What's more, dramatic changes in weight are not often necessary to improve your diabetes. Even losing 5 to 10 percent of your weight will help lower your blood sugar, reduce your blood pressure, improve your cholesterol levels, and increase your energy level.

Key strategies that can help you maintain a healthy body weight include:

- **Modifying your calories to meet your needs.** Your calorie needs will vary depending on your age, muscle mass, activity level, and genes.

- **Writing in a food journal.** Writing down your food intake can keep you focused on your goal and increase your intake of healthy foods.

- **Sticking to a plan of high-fiber, unprocessed food.** Eating high-fiber, unprocessed foods can decrease hunger and keep you feeling full longer.

- **Consuming the right amount of total calories from fat.** Keeping your fat intake low saves you calories and can decrease insulin resistance.

- **Eating adequate lean protein.** During weight loss, your muscle (your protein stores) are used up quickly. Maintaining your muscle mass will keep your metabolism high. To do this you will need to include enough protein in your diet.

- **Monitoring carbohydrate intake.** Too many carbohydrate foods increase blood sugar to a high degree. This leads to a need for more insulin, and when insulin increases in the body so does your ability to store excess calories into fat.

- **Drinking adequate water.** Drinking water and other noncalorie drinks like tea helps increase your metabolism and the feeling of fullness.

- **Avoiding medications that can cause weight gain** (see Chapter 3).

- **Exercising on a regular basis** (see Chapter 8).

- **Using behavior modification techniques** (see Chapter 7).

TO YOUR HEALTH

Even if you end up curing your diabetes by making healthy changes to your diet and losing weight, it is still wise to periodically check your blood sugar since diabetes can return later in life. Factors like aging, regaining weight, or being sick can cause diabetes to reappear. This is because prediabetes and type 2 diabetes have a significant genetic component.

Modifying Calories to Meet Energy Needs

It's hard to know how many calories are used on any given day due to the many individual and environmental factors that are involved. However, there is an easy way to estimate your calorie needs based on your weight and your activity level. Here is the formula in two easy steps:

1. Your weight in pounds × 10 = calories required to sustain (when resting without activity included)

2. Multiply calories required to sustain by an activity level factor

Activity level factors are estimates based on studies that determine energy expended during exercise. Here are the major categories:

- Sedentary or very light activity (sitting, sewing, cooking, reading, typing done most of the day): 1.2
- Semiactive (walking, dusting, playing golf done 30–60 minutes a day): 1.3
- Active (playing tennis, dancing, cycling, heavy housework done 60–90 minutes a day): 1.5
- Very active (playing sports like soccer, fast swimming, fast dancing, nonstop high-impact aerobic class done 90 minutes or more a day): 1.7+

An example of a semiactive person who weighs 160 pounds using these two calculations is:

$$160 \text{ lbs.} \times 10 = 1,600 \text{ calories}$$

$$1,600 \times 1.3 = 2,080 \text{ calories needed per day}$$

After using this formula to determine your everyday needs for weight maintenance, you can adjust your calorie consumption as needed to lose your weight.

How Many Calories Do You Need for Weight Loss?

To lose weight you will need to subtract calories from the usual amount of calories you need to maintain your weight. Every pound of body fat contains about 3,500 calories of stored energy. In order to lose a pound in a week, you need to eat about 500 fewer calories a day for seven days.

Putting the Numbers into Practice

In order to put a 1,600-calorie weight-loss diet into practice, you will need to monitor your carbohydrates as well as count calories. For the best results, meals should be spread out as evenly as possible throughout the day. Eating more often on a consistent basis can help keep your metabolism high and your blood sugar more level.

When you decide on a menu, add up calories and carbohydrates by looking them up in a calorie-carbohydrate counter book, or by using an electronic calculator. Some free electronic food calculators can be found online at www.choosemyplate.gov/supertracker-tools/supertracker.html and ndb.nal.usda.gov.

Staying Focused

Whether using example menus or devising your own menus, try writing down these foods along with their calories and carbohydrate grams. This activity will help you stay focused so that you can eventually change eating habits. However, if you find this is too much to do initially, don't worry. Just journaling what you eat once or twice a week can also help.

A group of researchers working with the *National Weight Control Registry survey* asked participants to record everything they ate at least one day, every week. The participants found that by doing this they eventually formed a habit of tracking their eating habits every day. Six months into the study, researchers found that the people who kept a daily food record had lost twice as much weight as everyone else in the study.

Presently, the registry has over 10,000 members. To join, you will need to have lost at least 30 pounds and have kept it off for at least one year. Go to nwcronline.com/join.aspx to learn more.

DEFINITION

The **National Weight Control Registry survey** is a research study that includes people who have lost at least 30 pounds and have kept it off for at least one year.

Planning Your Meals

Balancing carbohydrates, protein, and fat is the key to long-term success for maintaining healthy weight and good blood sugar control. About 50 to 60 percent of the diet should come from carbohydrates, 20 percent from protein, and 20 to 30 percent from fat. For the best blood sugar control and mental acuity, divide meals and snacks as evenly as possible throughout the day.

Protein

More protein is needed during weight loss to help prevent muscle loss. This is because when the body is deficient in calories it will use muscle tissue along with fat tissue to obtain calories for energy needs. If too much muscle is lost, you not only will be weaker, but your metabolism will decrease. Your body's muscle tissue burns up more calories than fat does.

Good sources for protein include fish, poultry, eggs, low-fat cheese, and lean meats. Two to three ounces of any of these foods, three times a day, should be sufficient. More than this is not good for your kidneys and can contribute to a significant amount of unneeded calories. The National Kidney Foundation suggests that diabetics keep their protein intake at about 15 percent of the total calories when not on a weight-reduction diet.

Each gram of protein contains 4 calories; however, some protein sources contain a higher fat content, such as prime rib, and will be higher in calories per ounce. In addition, the more fat in the protein source, the lower the actual protein grams will be per ounce.

To help keep calories lower and protein adequate, select skinless poultry and seafood instead of fatty meats. Food preparation plays a part; bake, broil, or roast instead of frying or sautéing with fats.

Dairy products such as yogurt or cottage cheese can be considered part of your total protein intake. One cup of yogurt or milk and ¼ cup of cottage cheese is equal to 1 ounce of meat, poultry, or fish.

✎ **TO YOUR HEALTH**

If you are a vegetarian, you can substitute beans and nuts for animal protein. One-half cup of beans or 2 tablespoons of nuts equals about the same amount of protein as 1 ounce of meat or poultry. However, beans have 15 grams of carbo-hydrates per ½ cup while meat has none.

Fat

Even though fat itself has a minimal impact on blood glucose levels, a diet high in *saturated fat* and *trans-fats* can lead to insulin resistance. Insulin resistance causes more blood sugar problems and decreased ability to lose weight. Foods high in saturated fat include cheese, butter, cream, red meat from grain-fed animals, poultry skin, and hydrogenated and partially hydrogenated fats. Foods high in trans-fats include most powdered coffee creamers, and some margarines and processed foods.

You can tell whether a product has trans-fats in it by reading the ingredient list. If there are partially hydrogenated vegetable oils listed, it has some trans-fats. This is true even if it states 0 trans-fats on the nutrition facts label. The USDA allows up to ½ gram of trans-fat in a single serving without requiring that it be labeled. If eating more than one serving, beware! You can be consuming a significant amount of trans-fats.

📖 **DEFINITION**

Saturated fat is a greasy or waxy solid fat which contains no double bonds in its fatty acid chain. This type of fat can cause coronary artery disease. **Trans-fats** are partially hydrogenated vegetable oils that are made solid by a chemical and heating process. These fats cause coronary artery disease to a degree higher than saturated fat.

The National Institutes of Health recommends that those wanting to lose weight should take in 7 percent or less of their calories from saturated fat, and 30 percent or less of their calories from polyunsaturated and monounsaturated fats.

Monounsaturated fats, also called omega-9 fatty acids, are liquid at room temperature and semisolid when refrigerated. These fats are less vulnerable to rancidity and protect against cardiovascular disease.

Polyunsaturated fats are fatty acids that remain liquid at both room and refrigerated temperatures. These fats include omega-3 and omega-6 fatty acids and protect against cardiovascular disease. In addition, research shows they may even help decrease insulin resistance when the ratio of omega-6 to omega-3 fatty acids is optimal—anywhere from 1:1 to 4:1. However, an excess amount of omega-6 fatty acids relative to omega-3 fatty acids can interfere with the action of omega-3 fatty acids and cause inflammation in the body.

Food sources high in omega-3, -6, and -9 fatty acids include the following:

- **Omega-3 fatty acids:** Fish, fish oil, flax seeds, chia seeds, hemp seeds, butternuts, and walnuts
- **Omega-6 fatty acids:** Safflower oil, cottonseed oil, sunflower oil, corn oil, soy oil, mixed vegetable oils, and more liquid types of margarines
- **Omega-9 fatty acids:** Almonds, peanuts, cashews, pecans, pistachios, avocadoes, olive oil, canola oil, and peanut oil

Eating healthy fats is a good choice, but you will still need to monitor the amounts. One gram of fat equals 9 calories, whether saturated or unsaturated fat. To keep your overall fat intake low, use seasonings such as natural fat-free butter-flavored powders, herbs, spices, vinegar, lemon juice, and small amounts of low-calorie salad dressings to flavor your food. Limit your consumption of butter, margarine, and oils. Use nonstick spray or nonstick cookware.

In order for you to maintain a fat intake of 20 to 30 percent of total calories, the grams of fat you eat depend on your total calorie level. For example, if you eat 2,200 calories with 20 percent of the calories from fat, you will get about 50 grams of fat for the day. Here is a list of how many fat grams you would take in for other calorie levels with a diet made up of 20 percent fat:

- 1,600 calories: 36 grams
- 1,800 calories: 40 grams
- 2,000 calories: 44 grams

Carbohydrates

The amount of carbohydrate foods you need is based on factors such as how much you exercise, your age, and your blood sugar levels. The more you exercise, the more carbohydrate foods you can consume without increasing your blood sugar. The older you are, the fewer carbohydrate foods you can consume before causing blood sugar problems.

Eating too many simple carbohydrates at one time increases blood sugar excessively. A prediabetic or a new type 2 diabetic will make more insulin in response to the high blood sugar. Producing extra insulin over a period of time can cause widely fluctuating sugar swings, and more fat storage.

A typical starting point for many adult diabetics is to eat about 45 to 60 grams of carbohydrates per meal and about 15 to 30 grams at a snack. However, this is not a magic number. To best determine if a specific amount of carbohydrate does not increase your blood sugar level, check your blood sugar two hours after eating. Preferably, blood sugar levels then should be less than or equal to 140 to 160.

Most of your carbohydrates should be unprocessed high fiber and low glycemic index. These types of carbohydrates help with controlling your hunger and are generally lower in calories. They include foods such as whole grains, vegetables, and fruits.

Fiber

One big reason people fail to lose weight is because they are still hungry after eating. Fiber plays a very important role in eliminating this problem. Fiber stays in the stomach longer and expands with fluids in the stomach. This causes a feeling of being full.

It is recommended that you get about 15 grams of fiber for every 1,000 calories consumed. For 1,500- to 3,000-calorie diets, the fiber range is between 22 and 44 grams per day.

The following table shows fiber content of some common foods.

	Amount	**Grams of Fiber**
High-fiber foods		
All-bran types of cereal	½ cup	8–14
Lentils	½ cup	7.8
Beans, pinto	½ cup	7.7
Beans, black	½ cup	7.5
Pear, fresh	1 medium	5.1
Moderate-fiber foods		
Figs, medium	2	3.8
Nuts, almonds	1 oz.	3.5
Apple (unpeeled)	1 medium	3.3
Apricots, dried	10 halves	2.6
Low-fiber foods		
Rice, white	½ cup	1–2
Bread, white	1 slice	1

Sources: USDA National Nutrient Database for Standard Reference, U.S. Department of Agriculture Research Service.

In developing a high-fiber meal plan, you will also want an adequate amount of lean protein and healthy fat at each meal. Just like fiber, both protein and fat help with satiety and blood sugar control. Here's an example of a high-fiber meal plan with 35 grams of fiber:

- **Breakfast:** ¾ cup unsweetened yogurt; ½ cup whole-grain, high-fiber cereal with 1 cup skim milk; ⅓ cup red grapes; 12 raw almonds

  Total fiber: 19 grams

- **Lunch:** 3 oz. cubed skinless baked chicken breast on one medium (10-inch) whole-wheat tortilla with ¼ sliced medium avocado and 2 TB. salsa; 1 cup celery/carrot sticks

  Total fiber: 9 grams

- **Dinner:** 3 oz. baked tilapia; one 8 oz. baked sweet potato topped with cinnamon; 2 oz. baked apple slices; spinach-pear salad with vinegar and oil; 6 raw walnuts

  Total fiber: 6 grams

- **Snack:** 1 cup cantaloupe with 1 cup sugar-free vanilla ice cream

  Total fiber: 1 gram

  Day's Total: 35 grams fiber

 RED FLAG

When increasing fiber in a diet, start gradually. A large, sudden increase could cause flatulence (gas) and bloating. In addition, drink an adequate amount of fluid to avoid a possible gastrointestinal obstruction. To prevent high blood sugar and excess calories, minimize drinks such as soda, juice, and drinks containing sugar.

Drink to Your Health

Drinking more water during the day can help with weight loss. Water not only helps to fill up your stomach and reduce hunger, but it also may speed up your metabolism.

Findings reported in the *Journal of Clinical Endocrinology and Metabolism* show that over the course of a year a person who increases his or her water consumption by 1 to 2 liters a day can lose more weight.

Men should consume about 96 ounces (of fluid a day, and women should drink about 64 ounces of fluid a day. Beverages like low-fat or skim milk, tea, and coffee without sugar or cream can also be included as part of the daily total. More than just a couple of beverages with caffeine can cause blood sugar to increase in some diabetics (more on this in Chapter 10).

Even though water is generally the best choice when consuming beverages, oftentimes not enough fluid gets consumed when only relying on water. To help reach your fluid needs, you may want to try some of these beverages. Calories and carbohydrate grams for each of the following is for 8 ounces:

- Diet cranberry juice cocktail (5 calories, 2 grams carbohydrates)
- Diet lemonade, iced tea, or punch, such as by Crystal Light (0–5 calories, 0–2 grams carbohydrates)
- Homemade lemonade sweetened with small amount of sugar substitute of your choice (0 calories, 0 grams carbohydrates)
- Iced or hot tea, plain or sweetened with small amount of sugar substitute of your choice (0 calories, 0 grams carbohydrates)
- Water with lemon wedges (0 calories, 0 grams carbohydrates)
- Diet sodas (limit to one a day)
- No-calorie to 5-calorie bottled waters (plain or fruit-flavored)

- Low-calorie or no-calorie drinks (0–5 calories, 0–2 grams carbohydrates), such as Diet Ocean Spray cranberry juice
- Diet hot cocoa mix (25 calories, 4 grams carbohydrates)

TO YOUR HEALTH

Watermelon punch can help quench your thirst, keep you hydrated, and add variety to your beverage choices. Combine 1 cup blended and strained watermelon, 3 cups water, 2 tablespoons lime juice, and the sugar substitute of your choice to taste. Each 8 -oz. serving has 15 calories and 14 grams carbohydrates.

Planning and Monitoring Your Diet

Now that you have an idea of the type of foods that you will be eating to lose weight, it's important that you plan for those foods. Planning is essential in order to lose weight successfully. Plan a week ahead and buy the groceries you will need in advance, then plan each day as you go through your week. An easy routine to develop is to sit down every night to plan the next day's menus. Check first to see what's available, then write your plan.

To start planning, it helps to use a menu pattern guide indicating how much protein, carbohydrates (starch, fruit, and dairy), and fat that you intend to have every day. The following table shows an example of a menu pattern guide for 1,600 calories.

Breakfast	Lunch	Dinner	Snack
2 oz. lean protein	3 oz. lean protein	3 oz. lean protein	
1 low-fat dairy		1 low-fat dairy	1 low-fat dairy
2 starches	2 starches	2 starches	2 starches
1 fruit			1 fruit
2 fats	2 fats	2 fats	
1 vegetable (optional)	2 vegetables	2 vegetables	

Writing a Meal Plan

Get a notebook and write in the day of the week at the top of the page. Across the top page, write the headings: Meals, Amount, Carbohydrate Grams, and Calories. Using a meal pattern, write in your planned breakfast, lunch, dinner, and snacks under the Meals heading. Under the headings titled Amount, Carbohydrate Grams, and Calories, write in quantity, carbohydrate grams and calories for each food.

You may not always have the exact type of food that your meal pattern guide indicates. This is not a problem; just substitute another food that has similar calories. For example, if you do not have fruit in your refrigerator, you can substitute a yogurt or slice of whole-grain bread. Whatever you use, though, make it add up to the specified calories you want for the day.

Reading Food Labels

To help you determine calories and carbohydrate grams, you will need to read food labels. Nutrition facts on food labels list the amount of carbohydrate content and calories per serving.

Here's an example label from a generic type of sugar-free ice cream, followed by some general tips for reading food labels.

- The nutrition facts on the label are based on the serving size; don't assume that one container equals one serving. This is often not the case. You may need to change the size of your serving in order to obtain the number of carbohydrate grams and calories that you want.

- Total carbohydrate grams on the label have subheadings for sugars, sugar alcohol, and fiber. These are part of what makes up the total carbohydrate grams. In the following example label there are 8g of sugar alcohol, 5g sugars, and 3g of dietary fiber. All the sugars are absorbed but not all the fiber and sugar alcohol.

Sugar-Free Ice Cream

Nutrition Facts:

Serving Size:	Servings per Container:
½ cup	13

Amount per Serving	**% Daily Value**
Calories 100	
Total Fat 0g	0%
Saturated Fat 0g	
Trans Fat 0g	
Cholesterol 10mg	1%
Sodium 75mg	3%
Total Carbohydrate 24g	8%
Dietary Fiber 3g	12%
Sugars 5g	
Sugar Alcohol 8g	
Protein 4g	7%

- Only half of fiber and sugar alcohol get absorbed; consequently, if a food contains more than 5 grams of fiber or sugar alcohol, subtract half from the total carbohydrate grams. This will give you the actual carbohydrate grams that will impact you. In the example label there is not enough fiber in this ice cream to worry about subtracting, but there is a significant amount of sugar alcohol, so if you want more precision, you would subtract 4 grams from the total carbohydrate of 24 to get 20 grams total carbohydrate that will impact you.

- The % Daily Value refers to how much of the recommended nutrient you are consuming, but these percentages are based a 2,000-calorie diet. So, some of the percent information will not apply to you.

Managing Insulin Needs as You Diet

When you reduce the number of carbohydrates and calories you
consume, you will also need to reduce your dosage of insulin
and/or medication. This is also true when you lose body weight.
At a lower body weight, your ability to use insulin is enhanced.

The amount of medication reduction will depend on how much
carbohydrates you reduced or how much weight you lost. The
more you reduce, the more pronounced the medication change
tends to be.

In order to determine how your body is responding to these
changes, check your blood glucose levels prior to and two hours
after you eat. If your blood sugar is lower than 70 prior to eating
or lower than 120 two hours after eating, eat a snack that con-
tains 15 grams of carbohydrates ($\frac{1}{2}$ cup juice, $\frac{1}{2}$ cup fruit, etc.).
Wait 15 minutes, and then recheck your blood sugar. If it's still
low, eat another 15-gram carbohydrate snack and retest after
15 minutes. Most often this is enough. If not, call your doctor
for advice about possible medication changes. You may need to
take a little less insulin or diabetic oral medication.

Strategies for Healthy Eating

Georgia flipped through the catalog until she saw a woman with light brown hair, blue eyes, and a pretty face. The woman weighed about 130 pounds and was 5 foot 6 inches tall and looked like Georgia—except that Georgia was 170 pounds. Georgia carefully tore out the page. She then cut around the outline of the woman with a scissors, and pasted the cutout figure onto the inside cover of her meal-planning notebook. Next, she placed a head photo of herself on top of the head of the paper-cutout woman.

Georgia thought, "There I am, the future Georgia!" Giddy with excitement at the prospect, she smiled and excitedly said, "I'll be able to wear my red dress again!"

Georgia is practicing visualization and positive thinking, one of the many ways that can help you achieve your weight and fitness goals. Other strategies include using behavior modification techniques, smart food management, and healthy food choices while dining out.

Visualization and Positive Thinking

Visualizing a healthy you can help you lose weight and eat better by keeping you motivated. When visualizing, focus on what you will feel and look like when you get to your desired weight. For the best results, do this on a daily basis.

In addition to cutting out a photo from a magazine like Georgia did to visualize her desired weight, you can try drawing an idealized self-portrait. The more detailed your drawing, the better. Draw where you will be and what outfit you will be wearing. To help see yourself as a healthy eater, you can also draw or cut out pictures of healthy food and make a collage. No matter what props you use to help you visualize, keep focused. Think long term. You are developing behaviors to last a lifetime.

TO YOUR HEALTH

Don't get bogged down by the everyday problems of living. They can take your focus away from what your goal is. To keep going when life gets tough can take a lot of positive thinking. To stay on target, read motivational books, attend classes about health, take time out for relaxation, and be around positive people.

Create a Living Space for Success

We may have the best eating intentions, but because of stressful events in our lives such as working too hard, getting stuck in traffic, or having a financial setback, we can weaken. An array of emotions can cause us to use old eating habits as a pacifier. When we are upset, our fight-flight hormones kick in and we go on autopilot. It becomes harder to make sound logical judgments.

So how can we stay focused and maintain our sanity? In addition to planning meals, learning how to navigate around work and mealtime environments can help.

Controlling Your Work Environment

I once had a work situation that caused me some sleep problems. It was several years ago when I drank coffee both in the morning and afternoon. The coffee worked well for me in the morning, but drinking it in the afternoon was causing havoc with my sleep. I tried to stopped, but could not seem to do it. Most days at around 2 P.M. I took a break in the cafeteria at the hospital where I worked. There was always a fresh pot of "free coffee," and despite my good intentions, every time I would give in to my cravings.

A couple years later, I started a new job where there was no longer accessible coffee. I immediately stopped drinking the coffee in the afternoon.

You don't need to wait until you get a new job before you change your eating habits. Here are some strategies to try:

- Don't keep unhealthy snacks at your desk.
- Decide what to eat prior to mealtime.
- Eat your own food and avoid unhealthy foods brought in by co-workers. If they insist you try their food, you can respond by saying, "I've already eaten," choose one bite only, or simply say, "No, thank you." In the case of having cake or other goodies for a co-worker's birthday, having just one bite might help you feel less deprived.
- Make it inconvenient to nibble on food by chewing gum, or drinking water or another noncaloric beverage.
- Bring portion-controlled healthy food to work.
- Don't let yourself get overly hungry by skipping meals.

Controlling Your Home Environment

The easiest place to overeat can be at home. We can eat in the living room in front of the TV, in our bedroom while lying in bed, in the kitchen while cooking a meal, and in the study while sitting in front of a computer. The more rooms you eat in, the more rooms you associate with eating. Just by being in a particular room will trigger your urge to eat! For example, you might associate watching TV with your dinner meal, or you might connect eating nuts and pretzels with working on the computer.

If you've already developed some of these habits, you will need to break them. A good way to do this is by substituting very low- or no-calorie foods for the usual foods you eat. These foods include noncaloric beverages and nonstarchy veggies like celery, cucumbers, and green peppers (with no dip!). Get rid of any high-calorie foods that you can't seem to eat in small quantities, such as cookies, nuts, chips, cake, and ice cream, and don't buy them anymore. If they're not in the house you can't eat them. It's a lot easier to talk yourself out of getting in the car and driving to get a treat than it is to reach into the freezer or cupboard.

I remember the time when I was alone in my apartment studying for an exam and there was a banana cake in the kitchen. I needed a break every one to two hours in order to stay awake, so I would get up to get a piece of cake at every break. By the end of the night I had eaten half of the cake! Here are some guidelines for avoiding mindless eating:

- Keep tempting foods out of the house.
- Arrange furniture you use a lot away from food areas. For example if your study desk and chair is in the kitchen, you may be more tempted to divulge in the leftovers stored in the refrigerator or nuts in the cupboard.
- Have healthy snacks at your disposal, such as raw vegetables, fresh fruit, and noncaloric beverages. Cut up vegetables and fruit and put into single-serve containers and you may find that you will be more likely to eat them.
- Plan what you will be eating ahead of time and stick with your meal plan.

• Do not watch TV, read, or sit anywhere but the dinner table while eating meals or higher-caloric foods such as cheese, breads, chips, etc.

Food Management and Behavior Modification

Managing your food includes controlling portions, shopping, preparing food, dealing with hunger, and overcoming bad habits.

Replace Bad Habits with Good Ones

Habits simplify our lives and save us energy and stress. We don't have to think, we do. The secret is to replace a bad habit with a good one. To do this, plan a new good habit, start it, practice it, and provide incentives along the way. Here are ways to implement these four major steps:

1. **Plan.** Take a few days to analyze your behaviors, and decide which behavior to change. For example, it might be to change your snacking behavior in the afternoon.

2. **Start a new habit in place of the bad habit.** Replace that behavior with a noneating activity, such as taking a shower, going for a walk, playing tennis, going shopping, or working in the garden.

3. **Repeat the new behavior.** Plan the new behavior into your everyday schedule to make this happen. If something interferes with your new behavior being carried out, have a backup plan. For example, if your new behavior is to play tennis in the afternoon and it rains, substitute the tennis with something like walking in the mall or shopping. An eating behavior that becomes easier with repetition is eating more vegetables and fruit instead of refined starchy or sugary foods. See more in the next section on how refined foods and sugar make hunger worse.

4. **Provide incentives along the way.** Use both external and internal incentives. An external incentive is to reward yourself for your new behavior by doing something you love, such as taking a bubble bath, listening to music, or having your hair fixed. An inner incentive comes from a feeling of accomplishment and doing the right thing. To help assure yourself of providing incentives, write down your new behavior in a notebook or your meal-planning book. Next to your new behavior write in a daily incentive.

Keeping Hunger in Check

If you are overly hungry prior to a meal, try drinking a large glass of water or other noncaloric beverage. If you still feel hungry 15 minutes later, eat foods like raw, nonstarchy watery veggies like cucumbers, celery, and green peppers.

Eating too many simple carbohydrate foods like refined breads, rice, and desserts can cause more hunger. When these foods are consumed, the blood sugar rises to a high level requiring the body will need to make (or inject) extra insulin in order to compensate. With the extra insulin your blood sugar will drop even lower than prior to eating in just a couple of hours and you will be hungry again.

Also, you will want to avoid skipping meals to avoid hunger. Your body needs nourishment every 3 to 4 hours. Eat meals that are balanced and contain a protein like chicken, fish, or cottage cheese, a high-fiber unprocessed carbohydrate like whole-grain bread or pasta, and a healthy snack like nuts or part of an avocado.

Food Preparation

Don't snack while cooking meals unless you only eat raw, nonstarchy vegetables like celery or carrots. If you have to taste the food, put only a tiny dab or mini-bite-sized piece on a spoon to taste.

Fix only enough food to eat, unless you need to take your meal to work the next day. Prior to sitting down to eat your meal, portion out the food you will be taking to work and place it in a storage container.

> ### TO YOUR HEALTH
>
> To prevent yourself from overeating, eat slowly. Chew your food thoroughly and put your utensils down in between bites. Stop eating for a minute or two during your meal to reflect on how the food tastes. If you're eating with someone else, talk between bites. By the end of the meal, you will feel full and be less likely to overeat later.

Portion Control

Portion control can be easy when you make your food ahead of time and use sandwich bags or plastic containers. For example, if you want exactly 30 grams of carbohydrates and 160 calories of pasta, then measure ²/₃ cup of pasta to put into a baggie. Freeze any extra portions. Preportioned leftovers are great foods to take to work.

To get your calories and carbohydrate counts right, measure portions with a measuring cup and spoons, or use a scale. It's too easy to underestimate what you actually eat. After you are accustomed to what a specific portion looks like, it will be easier for you to estimate food quantities when you don't have measuring devices available, such as at a restaurant or at a friend's house. Another guide to use when eating out is the MyPlate or GI Plate method found in Chapter 4.

Smart Shopping

Shop from a list and avoid buying anything but what is on your list. Your food list should be organized into food sections: dairy, fresh vegetables, fresh fruits, fresh lean protein, frozen foods, and dry products.

When you pass by the food sampling stations in the store, do not let your defense down. To keep your defenses higher, do not go to the store when you are hungry or tired.

Finally, read food labels in order to choose the healthiest options (see Chapter 6 for a sample food label). Check carbohydrate content, calories, fat, and protein per serving. Also, look at the ingredient list. The food ingredients are listed in order of highest percent to lowest percent of the total food composition of that item.

More Strategies for Success

Maximize your chance of success by using as many ways or strategies that you can. The more you can do the better your ability will be to keep your weight where you want it. Strategies for weight management for individuals who have lost weight and kept it off include being physically active, checking their weight almost every day, joining a weight management program, being in the company of healthy people, and seeking out professional help when needed.

Stay Active

Increasing activity can help burn more calories, keep you happier by increasing your *serotonin* level, increase your self-esteem, and improve your blood sugar. See Chapter 8 on exercise and diabetes.

 DEFINITION

Serotonin is a brain chemical (neuro-transmitter) that makes us happy and contented.

Weigh Yourself Every Day

If you don't have a scale, buy one. It can help you improve your focus and weight status. Individuals who have lost weight and kept it off in the National Weight Control Registry survey mentioned earlier weighed themselves almost daily. Weighing yourself often gives feedback on your weight status and helps reinforce your mission of staying healthy and fit. Try weighing yourself at least a couple times a week or more often to see if helps keep you more focused on your goals.

Join a Weight Management Program

Some individuals use their own weight-loss plan, but joining a good weight management program may be beneficial. Whether you join a support group or go solo, implement your program for six months or longer. Statistically, new eating habits have an increased rate of success the longer the habit is practiced.

Get Help from a Pro

Seek out professional help if you have tried everything but are still unable to lose weight. You may have a thyroid deficiency or you may be on a medication that causes weight gain. Your doctor can check your thyroid function, or prescribe a substitute medication for one that may be causing weight gain. In addition, he or she may prescribe medications designed to help you lose weight.

If you are dealing with extreme emotional problems that are preventing you from changing your eating habits, consider seeing a mental health professional. Counselors can help you with talk therapy and, if needed, prescribe medications.

RED FLAG

If you receive an antidepressant medication, make sure that weight gain is not a side effect. Ask your doctor about any side effects of the medication you take. Many of the medications taken for depression can cause weight gain. Some antidepression medications, however, such as Wellbutrin, can help lift depression and aid with weight loss.

Be in the Company of Healthy People

Have you ever heard the statement "whoever you live with you become like"? It's true! Studies have shown that we tend to mimic the people we spend the majority of our time with. If you want to lose weight and stay healthy, spend more time with people who are healthy and at their right body weight.

Dining Out

Dining out is often associated with weight gain. Studies have shown that people who like to patronize restaurants overeat and are more likely to be overweight. This is understandable, since portions are larger and contain higher quantities of fat and con-centrated carbohydrates than foods served at home where you have control.

To gain more control ask your waiter to have your order pre-pared a certain way. In order to estimate portion size at a restaurant, measure foods you eat at home. To be better able to know if food has fat or added sugars, notice how such foods look, taste, and, feel. If you see food with an oily film on it, you will know that some type of fat was added. If you are unsure, touch the food with your fingers and then rub your fingers together to see if they become oily. Added sugars are harder to spot in foods, but you can do a taste test to make sure. If you are served food that you don't want, don't be afraid to ask for a replacement.

Keeping good blood sugar control and maintaining a healthy weight when dining out can be easier if you follow these tips:

- Avoid skipping meals prior to eating out.
- Avoid having a low blood sugar. Waiting to take your insulin just before the meal is served.
- If you take a medication that increases your insulin level, have a healthy snack prior to leaving for the restaurant.
- Count your carbohydrate servings. If there are too many carbohydrates, ask to replace some of the rice, potatoes, or pasta with nonstarchy vegetables or cottage cheese, options that don't require special preparation.
- Eat slowly, relax, and chew your food thoroughly. You will enjoy the meal more and it will be easier for you to eat less.
- Ask for a take-home box or bag prior to eating. Portion out part of the meal so you won't be tempted to eat the whole entrée.

Breakfast

Breakfast foods that will help you lose weight include coffee, tea, low-fat milk, low-fat plain yogurt, cottage cheese, eggs, egg substitutes, fresh fruit, cold and hot cereals, and whole-grain toast. Ask to have items prepared without oils, margarine, or butter.

Breakfast foods to avoid include biscuits, gravy, syrups, croissants, omelets cooked in butter or oil, high-fat cheese, bacon, sausage, and white flour pancakes and waffles.

Dinner and Lunch

Protein foods for dinner and lunch can include grilled fish, chicken, cottage cheese, and lean meats. Ask for meat, poultry, and fish to be cooked without added fat.

Starchy foods include baked potatoes, rice, and pasta. Avoid butter, sour cream, sauces, or oils. Be sure to monitor your portion size for good blood sugar control.

Acceptable side dishes are vegetables, beans, corn, fruit, broth soups, and salads. Ask for them to be prepared without added fats or sauces.

Bread choices can include corn or plain flour tortillas, whole-grain and sourdough breads, and flat bread. However, you may need to limit or omit these if you are already at your carbohydrate limit for the meal.

Foods to avoid include cream-based soups, gravies, cheese, sauces, bacon, crunchy chow mein noodles, dressings, biscuits, deep-fried foods, casseroles, croutons, and breaded products.

Understanding Menu Terminology

Choosing the healthier entrée becomes more challenging if you are not familiar with menu terminology. The following table shows some of the common menu phrases for lower- and higher-fat foods.

Healthier Choice (lower fat)	Heavier Choice (higher in fat)
Barbecued	Alfredo
Broiled	*Au gratin* (with cheese)
Charbroiled	*Béarnaise*
Marinara	Cream sauce
Tomato sauce	Newburg
Poached	Creamed
Steamed	Marinated in butter

Whenever you are eating away from home, continue to make the meal fit into your meal pattern. If it helps, take your diary meal plan with you (see Chapter 6).

Social Eating

Social events can trigger binge eating. There are a lot of happy memories and special foods associated with the holidays. For example, I often hear statements such as, "Thanksgiving can't be Thanksgiving unless there is the pecan pie and creamed marshmallow sweet potato casserole." If you can eat just one or two bites of some of these foods without being triggered to eat more no problem, however if you know you can't stop at just one bite, you might want to avoid the higher calorie goodies entirely, Even if you skip the pecan pie and sweet potato casserole, you can still happily connect with your friends or family. It just takes a little redirection. Here are some tips.

Don't Arrive Hungry

Whether going to a friend's house for dinner or to a party during the holidays, don't arrive too hungry. Do not skip meals beforehand, and, if needed, have a light snack prior to arriving. It is easy to overeat when you're hungry.

Visualize Healthy Eating

It's also easy to overindulge when you're at a social gathering and you lose focus. To help prevent going on autopilot, eat a healthy snack and then visualize not overeating at the party.

While at home, close your eyes and focus on who you will meet and what you will be eating. If you know that there will be vegetables and diet soda at your get-together, then see yourself nibbling on veggies and sipping diet soda.

Make Some of the Food

If you are going to a friend's house, offer to bring a healthy side dish or dessert and some diet soda along. Consume small portions of foods that are higher in calories and larger portions of foods that are lower in calories.

Be a Natural

Don't make a big deal about your new eating habits at social events. Announcing that you are cutting down on calories because you need to lose weight sets you up for scrutiny and judgment, which can make you feel inferior. Also, people may tend to sabotage your efforts (even though they may not mean to). When you make a change it can make some people feel uncomfortable and because of this, they may even encourage you to eat.

The most important reason to get together with friends and family is to enjoy each other's company, not to talk about your healthy choice.

Exercise and Diabetes

Pete fumbled in the dark to find the off button of his alarm clock. He thought, "It can't be time to get up already." Then he remembered that he had made plans to meet his girlfriend, Nancy, at the gym by 6 A.M. They had made a pact to try to lose weight. He and Nancy planned to work out together on Monday, Wednesday, and Friday mornings before work. Pete was just diagnosed with prediabetes, and hoped the exercise, along with some weight loss, might make his condition go away.

Well, Pete will be happy to know that he might be right! Anyone with diabetes can benefit from exercise and from loss of excess weight. The benefits include better blood sugar control, burning excess body fat, improved circulation, reduced stress, increased energy and muscle strength, and protection from heart disease and nerve and eye damage.

But certain precautions should be taken when starting a new exercise regimen. This chapter will help you use exercise to help improve your diabetes.

Considerations for Exercising with Diabetes

Before starting an exercise program, check with your doctor. If you are taking insulin or if you have nerve damage, eye problems, uncontrolled blood pressure, or cardiovascular disease, some kinds of exercise can make your problems worse. Activities such as lifting weights can make eye problems worse. You may be advised to walk or do tai chi. On the other hand, walking or running with nerve damage in your feet can cause pressure sores or foot injuries, so you may be advised to swim or do exercise on a stationary bike.

Using Insulin

Another consideration to take into account prior to exercise is the type of diabetic medication that you are taking. If you take insulin or a medication that increases the secretion of insulin, you will need to test your blood sugar prior to exercising and again right after exercising in order to prevent low blood sugar. Here are some guidelines that can help:

- If your blood sugar is 100 or lower prior to exercise, you may need a small carbohydrate snack before you exercise, such as a piece of fruit or one light yogurt .

- If your blood sugar is 100 to 250 prior to exercise, generally no changes need to be made.

- If your blood sugar is 250 or higher, test your ketones with your meter. Ketones are substances that build up when your body breaks down fat for energy and your cells can't use blood sugar as a fuel. This happens when there isn't enough insulin to transport blood sugar into the cells. If you have excess ketones, wait to exercise until your test kit indicates a low level of ketones in your urine.

RED FLAG

The presence of ketones leads to dehydration. If you exercise while dehydrated, you will produce even more ketones, causing even more dehydration and elevated blood sugar that can lead to diabetic ketoacidosis. Common symptoms prior to ketoacidosis include rapid breathing, dry mouth, flushed face, nausea, or stomach pain. Diabetic ketoacidosis is a life-threatening condition if left untreated. See Chapter 1 for more details.

Eating Prior to Exercise

If you are not taking insulin or insulin-secreting medications, eating prior to exercise in order to avoid hypoglycemia is generally not needed. However, if you take insulin or a secretagogue (an insulin-secreting medication) like glyburide and don't need to lose weight, add a carbohydrate snack before exercising. If you start out with a "safe" blood sugar prior to exercise, follow this protocol to prevent a low blood sugar during and after exercise:

- For moderate exercise of less than 30 minutes, no additional carbohydrates are needed.

- For moderate exercise of an hour, eat an additional 15 grams of carbohydrates (½ cup of juice, one small piece of fruit, one light yogurt, two rice cakes, six jelly beans, or four to five Lifesaver candies).

- For an hour of strenuous exercise, eat a carbohydrate food with 30 grams of carbohydrate prior to exercise. Examples include 1 cup juice, one large piece of fruit, two rice cakes with 1½ tablespoons of pure fruit jam, four small sugar-free cookies, or five vanilla wafers. For more than an hour of moderate or strenuous exercise, you will need to take additional snacks with you while exercising depending on the time and intensity you expect to exercise.

Moderate exercise might include these examples:

- Dancing to a fast waltz for 30 minutes
- Walking 2 miles in 30 minutes
- Performing water aerobics for 30 minutes
- Shooting baskets for 30 minutes

Strenuous exercise might involve the following:

- Walking very fast uphill (such as on a treadmill) for 60 minutes or more
- Running 4 miles in 30 minutes or less
- Swimming moderately fast to fast laps for 45 minutes or more
- Playing soccer for 60 minutes or more

Adjusting Insulin Before Exercise

If you are overweight and are taking insulin or insulin-secreting medications, check with your doctor about decreasing your short-acting insulin dosage by 10 to 30 percent on exercise days.

In order to determine exactly how much less insulin or medication you will need, check your blood sugar before and after exercising. If you are able to stay in the range of 100 to 180 blood sugar before and after exercise, you are in a safe zone. If your blood sugar is higher you decreased your dosage too much. If your blood sugar is too low, you probably took too much insulin. As you monitor your blood sugar, keep in mind that your blood glucose can continue to drop for hours after exercising. If an exercise routine is new for you, you may need to check your blood sugar more than just before and after exercise.

Monitoring High Blood Sugar with Strenuous Exercise

Strenuous exercise can result in high blood sugar if you are not conditioned to that type of exercise. The fight-flight hormone, cortisol, can stimulate the release of glycogen from liver and muscles. Glycogen is a form of starch energy that turns into blood sugar. If this happens, monitor your blood sugar. Do not give yourself more insulin, immediately, but if your blood sugar is over 300 mg/dL after exercise call your doctor for advice.

Like moderate exercise, blood glucose levels can continue to drop for hours after exercise and intense exercise prolongs the glucose-lowering effect. Check your blood sugar for every couple of hours for up to eight hours after strenuous activity in the beginning.

Reducing the Risk of Low Blood Sugar

If you take too much insulin or insulin secretagogue like glyburide (an insulin-secreting medication) without eating any food, you can develop hypoglycemia (low blood sugar). This happens most frequently when you have exercised for prolonged periods of time but it can also happen for shorter periods of exercise.

TO YOUR HEALTH

During exercise, it can be difficult to know when you're hypoglycemic because the usual warning signs such as sweating, rapid heartbeat, and shaking can be mistaken for normal exercise responses. This is why it is so important to check your blood sugar levels before and after exercising, especially when starting a new exercise program.

The reason low blood sugar is more likely to occur in diabetic people who are not in good physical shape and who exercise sporadically is because the usual replenishment of muscle and liver glycogen stores that builds up with consistent regular exercise is not fully effective yet.

If you are starting a new exercise routine, you need to check blood sugar before and after exercise. You should periodically check your blood sugar for up to 24 hours. If you are planning on doing a particular type of exercise on a regular basis, experiment with the exercise at the same time of day for at least three to four days before you decrease your blood sugar monitoring.

Exercising Safely

To prevent complications with blood sugar while exercising, you should take some precautions:

- Carry some quickly absorbed carbohydrates, such as fruit juice or hard candy.
- Wear an ID tag to identify you as diabetic.
- Protect your feet by wearing shoes and socks that fit properly.
- If you experience severe shortness of breath, or a sharp pain or pressure anywhere in your body, stop exercising.
- Avoid exercising when your insulin is at its peak level. For peak insulin times, see Chapter 3 on medications.
- Be consistent with exercise and meal times, have a regular schedule.
- Even though you can decrease the amount of insulin used prior to exercise, don't skip insulin. It can result in ketoacidosis.
- Drink adequate fluid to prevent dehydration (see the following section).

The Importance of Hydration

Even with slight dehydration of less than 2 percent, exercise becomes more difficult and possibly dangerous. Consequently, it's important to drink water or other acceptable beverages even if you are not sure if you are dehydrated. It's better to be a little overhydrated prior to exercise than dehydrated. The negative effects of dehydration include increased heart rate, decrease in oxygen-carrying capacity, and an increase in body temperature.

When you exercise, your body loses fluid through sweat to cool itself. Depending on the conditions such as intensity of exercise, temperature, and how long you exercise, varying amounts of fluid are lost. On a warm day, it is not uncommon to lose up to 16 ounces of water through sweat while exercising for an hour.

RED FLAG

If your blood sugar is elevated, it can cause the excess sugar along with water to spill into the urine. This can cause significant dehydration if fluid is not replaced. If your blood sugar is high, replace fluid by drinking an extra 16 to 24 ounces of water.

The recommended amount of fluid to drink prior to exercising for 30 minutes to 1 hour is 16 to 24 ounces. You might need more water if the temperature is warmer or you perspire heavily. You can tell if you got enough water by examining the color of your urine. If it is a pale yellow, you're well hydrated; if it is dark yellow, you are probably dehydrated.

A person typically needs about 10 to 12 cups per day of fluid. In addition to water, you can drink low-calorie fruit-flavored drinks, weak caffeinated tea, decaffeinated tea and coffee, and up to two cups of regular coffee or strong tea. For more ideas, see Chapter 6.

How Much Exercise?

The American Diabetes Association (ADA) advises diabetics to perform at least 150 minutes a week of moderately intense physical activity, such as walking, swimming, biking, dancing, and water aerobics. For weight loss, they suggest exercising for at least 210 minutes of moderate to intense exercise every week.

For maximum blood sugar benefits, leave no more than two days between exercise sessions. The effect aerobic exercise has on increasing insulin sensitivity only last 24 to 72 hours. For the most optimal health and weight benefits, exercise every day for at least 30 minutes each session.

What Type of Exercise?

The three major types of exercise are strength building, aerobic, and stretching. Even though all of these are not meant for everyone, at least one of these can benefit you.

Strength Building

Strength-building exercise (also called resistance training) can tone muscles, improve strength, and increase muscle mass. The more muscle you have, the higher your metabolism will be. In addition, resistance exercises have been shown to increase insulin sensitivity. These exercises include using free and machine weights, or doing calisthenics such as push-ups, sit-ups, and chin-ups. Strength-building exercise is not recommended for those with nerve damage, eye problems, uncontrolled blood pressure, or cardiovascular disease.

Do five minutes of aerobic exercise prior to starting strength-building exercises. It is also suggested that you do strength-building exercise that involve all major muscle groups two or more days a week.

Aerobic Exercise

Aerobic exercise includes walking, swimming, or cycling. It can improve your blood sugar and insulin sensitivity, start slowly and gradually increase speed and duration to prevent injury. After you are conditioned, you will find aerobic exercise can increase your energy level and endurance throughout the day.

If you need to lose or maintain weight, aerobic exercise is the most efficient way to do it. It is also an excellent way to increase circulation and oxygen to all parts of the body. It helps boost serotonin levels in the brain and gives a feeling of well-being, which can help you stay positive and focused on your weight and blood sugar goals. Finally, aerobic exercise can help prevent cardiovascular disease, cancer, and kidney disease.

Stretching Exercises

Stretching can help improve flexibility, decrease muscle pain, and help prevent injury. Before you start make sure you are stretching safely. To help prevent injury, follow these guidelines:

- Don't stretch as a warm-up. Stretching cold muscles can injure them. Before stretching, do some walking, jogging, or biking for at least five minutes.
- Stretch muscles and joints that you routinely use, and include both sides of your body.
- Hold each stretch; don't bounce. Bouncing can leave muscle tears that tighten and make the muscle even less flexible.
- Stretch just to ease tension; it should not hurt.
- For best results, stretch every day.

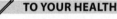

TO YOUR HEALTH

If you want to run a marathon, participate in a triathlon, or run a 5K, seek the help of a trainer with diabetes experience. You will need to test your blood sugar more often and closely follow the directions of your trainer.

Getting Into the Exercise Habit

Exercise is one of the best ways to control the symptoms of diabetes and improve your overall health. It can increase your energy level and insulin sensitivity, normalize your weight, improve your mood, and help prevent cardiovascular disease and cancer. In addition, it can improve your sleep, digestion, immunity, and bone density.

With all of these benefits, why do so many of us not exercise? Here's what I hear from my clients: "I don't have enough time with my work schedule ... I exercise enough at work ... I can't because my foot hurts ... I feel and look fat in gym clothes." The list of excuses goes on. The truth is we can find time to exercise, and even a small amount of exercise can make a difference. Here are some suggestions on how to increase your activity level without even going to the gym:

- Park your car at the far end of the parking lot.
- Walk up and down stairs instead of taking an elevator.
- Instead of meeting friends for coffee, meet for a walk.
- Take exercise breaks at work.

Try to set aside some time three to four times a week to go to the gym, a pool, or outdoors for exercise. Find a pleasant and convenient setting, and determine what exercise appeals to you. Set a schedule and commit to exercise as part of your usual routine. Exercise habits can be hard to develop, so you might have to develop a strategy to get you started. For example, arrange to go to the gym with a friend.

It's also a good idea to have a backup plan for when you are not able to get to the gym. If your babysitter just called and can't watch your kids while you're at the gym, put on a DVD exercise program or a CD of peppy music and dance or move to the music. In fact, have your kids join you! They will have a great time and all of you will get exercise.

Our lives are full of challenges. Don't let them deter you from your goals of taking care of yourself. Stay focused. Imagine yourself as a healthy person at an ideal body weight. Then make it happen!

Supplements for Diabetes

Gladys came toward the nurses' station and saw Roxanne. Gladys exclaimed, "Roxanne, you were right, the fenugreek does help control appetite! I put some in my soup yesterday and after that I didn't feel hungry until supper time."

"That's great," Roxanne replied. "I'm glad it helped. Did you decrease your insulin before using the fenugreek?"

"No," Gladys admitted. "I didn't really think it would make much of a difference, but now that I think of it, my blood sugar reading was low right before dinner."

"That makes sense; the herb can decrease carbohydrate absorption and intensify the action of hypoglycemic medications," Roxanne replied.

"It's amazing how many interactions can occur with diet, supplements, and medications!" said Gladys.

Gladys and Roxanne are not alone in using alternative medicines. According to surveys, at least 75 percent of the population use complementary and alternative therapies. This chapter will focus on herbal and vitamin-mineral supplementation because of their use in helping alleviate the symptoms of diabetes.

Should You Take a Supplement?

A supplement is a product that is taken by mouth as a pill, capsule, tablet, powder, or liquid. It contains one or more dietary ingredients such as vitamins, minerals, herbs, amino acids, or fiber, and it is also labeled as a dietary supplement.

The label on a dietary supplement container may make a claim concerning health, nutrient content, or structure/function. These claims describe a relationship between food components in the product that reduce the risk of a health-related condition.

 RED FLAG

In the United States, dietary supplements are not approved for safety or effectiveness before they reach the consumer. It is only once a supplement is marketed that the FDA can determine that a product is unsafe and restrict its use. Therefore, it is important for the consumer to investigate a supplement prior to using.

Not All Supplements Are Equal

Dietary supplements can differ depending on manufacturing techniques and where the raw products were harvested. Some are purer, more potent, or fresher than others. Some may even contain harmful filler chemicals. One good way to check products for efficacy and reliability is to go online to one of these websites:

- Tips for the savvy supplement user: www.fda.gov/Food/ DietarySupplements/default.htm

- Tips for the older supplement user: www.fda.gov/Food/DietarySupplements/Consumerinformation/ucm110493.htm
- FDA MedWatch: www.fda.gov/medwatch
- National Center for Complementary and Alternative Medicine: nccam.nih.gov
- Office of Dietary Supplements: www.ods.od.nih.gov
- U.S. Pharmacopeial Convention: www.usp.org
- Health fraud awareness: www.fda.gov/forconsumers/protectyourself/healthfraud/default.htm

Why Use a Supplement?

Ask yourself these questions before buying any supplement (and again, be sure to discuss with your doctor):

- Why do I want to use a product?
- What do I want to achieve?
- What is the best source of information about the product?
- How do I add a supplement?
- How long before I see an effect?
- How much does it cost?
- How will it affect my other medications? Ask your doctor prior to using any supplements.
- Can eating a healthy diet do the same thing I want to accomplish without adding a supplement?

TO YOUR HEALTH

Supplements are made to complement the diet, not replace eating certain foods. Whole foods contain a variety of micronutrients, whereas a supplement will not be a whole food. For example, if you take vitamin C you will get only vitamin C, but if you eat a raw green pepper, you will not only get a lot of vitamin C, but also fiber and phytochemicals as well—all of which will boost your overall health.

Vitamins and Minerals to Help Lower Blood Sugar

Some supplements, taken in the right amount and for the right reason can be advantageous. According to research, the vitamins and minerals most likely to improve blood sugar levels or to help alleviate complications of diabetes include vitamin B-12, vitamin B-1, magnesium, chromium, and alpha lipoic acid. But a word of caution: just because some of these nutrients may be helpful for some they may not be helpful for you. The key to good nutrition and health is balance. Too much of a good thing can causes the body to be imbalanced.

The B Vitamins

In order to maintain good health we need all the B-complex vitamins, including thiamine, riboflavin, niacin, pyridoxine, folic acid, biotin, pantothenic acid, inositol, choline, and B-12. However, you may need more of two of these B vitamins if you take metformin, a common oral diabetic medication. Metformin can use up or decrease the absorption of vitamin B-12 and vitamin B-1.

Vitamin B-12. Vitamin B-12 helps prevent anemia, dementia, and possibly heart disease. As we age, it gets harder for our bodies to absorb this vitamin. Many older people also experience decreased acidity in their stomach. This makes it more difficult to absorb vitamin B-12 and other nutrients. Other high-risk groups for a vitamin B-12 deficiency include individuals who have a gastric bypass, or who have gastrointestinal disorders such as celiac disease or inflammatory bowel.

Food sources high in B-12 include eggs, meat, poultry, seafood, and dairy products.

Supplementing your diet with vitamin B-12 can be beneficial if you use metformin or a diuretic. Recommended doses are 25 to 50 micrograms a day. To find out if you need a supplement higher than the recommended dose, ask your doctor.

Thiamine (Vitamin B-1). Thiamine or vitamin B-1 can also be affected by metformin. Studies have shown that thiamine passes through the kidneys and is not reabsorbed back into the blood as well as it is for people without diabetes. Thiamine is used by the body to break down sugars in the diet and it can help correct nerve and heart disorders.

Food sources high in thiamine include eggs, lean meats, nuts and seeds, peas, and whole grains.

Thiamine comes in fat- and water-soluble forms. The water-soluble dose for those with a mild deficiency is 5 to 30 milligrams per day and up to 300 milligrams a day for a severe deficiency. Benfotiamine, a fat-soluble form of thiamine, is often recommended for many diabetics since it is better absorbed than the water-soluble form. The best dose of Benfotiamine for neuropathy (nerve damage) is 300 milligrams a day.

B-Complex. One option for obtaining thiamine and vitamin B-12 is to take a B-complex vitamin supplement. The advantage of taking a complex supplement is that there is a better nutrient balance. Balance is important because too much of any one vitamin or mineral can cause deficiencies in other nutrients—all nutrients work best when balanced. A complete B-complex supplement will include thiamine, riboflavin, niacin, pyridoxine, folic acid, biotin, pantothenic acid, inositol, choline, and B-12.

A suggested dose is to take a half serving of B-complex vitamins containing 250 to 500 percent of the RDA (recommended daily allowance).

Magnesium

Magnesium is the fourth most abundant mineral in the body. It helps regulate blood sugar levels, is involved in energy metabolism and protein synthesis, and promotes normal blood pressure. Populations with the highest levels of magnesium are found to have the lowest risk of diabetes.

Magnesium is absorbed in the small intestine and excreted through the kidneys. People with insulin resistance tend to have less of this mineral because they excrete more in their urine. This is especially true when the blood sugar levels become elevated or if you are taking a diuretic.

Studies have shown that diabetics who take supplemental magnesium every day have a decreased fasting glucose and less neuropathy. The recommended daily allowance for magnesium is 400 milligrams a day, but surveys have shown that Americans do not get enough magnesium. This may be related to the use of medications such as diuretics, antibiotics, and drugs used to treat cancer, in addition to poorly controlled blood sugar.

 RED FLAG

Taking over 800 milligrams of magnesium a day is not recommended. Too much magnesium can cause loose stools and diarrhea.

Foods high in magnesium are whole grains, nuts, legumes, spinach, yogurt, milk, and salmon.

A supplement of between 100 and 350 milligrams a day can be of benefit if you have diabetes and/or use a diuretic.

Chromium

Several studies have found that chromium increases insulin sensitivity and may help in the reduction of carbohydrate cravings. A deficiency can cause decreased insulin sensitivity, depression, and decreased lean muscle mass.

Chromium deficiency can become an issue with extreme exercise, physical trauma, burns, chronic stress, high blood sugar levels, and aging. In the United States, the dietary guideline for chromium is between 25 and 35 micrograms per day. Eating foods high in vitamin C along with foods or supplements containing chromium can improve the absorption.

Foods high in chromium include dark chocolate, beef and beef liver, chicken, dairy products, eggs, seafood, whole grains, and nuts.

Since chromium is a trace nutrient you should keep the dose at or under 50 micrograms per day, or better yet, eat more foods high in chromium.

Alpha Lipoic Acid

Alpha lipoic acid (ALA) is a vitamin-like substance that can help improve blood sugar levels by assisting in the breakdown of carbohydrates for energy. ALA also acts as an anti-inflammatory and antioxidant agent which decreases cell damage. Finally, ALA is noted for its effect on diabetic neuropathy (nerve damage). ALA can help improve function and conduction of the neurons.

Good food sources of ALA include brewer's yeast, liver, heart, kidney, tomato, spinach, broccoli, and potatoes. If your diet is adequate in ALA but you are still having problems with neuropathy, ask your doctor about taking ALA to improve your symptoms.

If you have neuropathy, 600 to 1,200 milligrams a day may be beneficial. Ask your doctor about this or other medications used to treat neuropathy.

Fiber Supplements

Dietary fiber consists of nonstarchy polysaccharides called cellulose and chitin, as well as other plant particles such as dextrins, inulin, ligin, pectin, beta-glucans, and oligosaccharides. As a rule, fiber is not digested or absorbed. It passes relatively intact through the stomach, small intestine, and colon. It doesn't contain notable calories or carbohydrate value that can add to weight gain and blood sugar problems.

Fiber is grouped into two categories: soluble and insoluble. Soluble fiber is viscous and sticky (like pectin and guar gum), and insoluble fiber is hard (like wheat bran and celery stalks). Both of these fibers help us feel more full after eating them, but soluble fiber has the biggest impact on lowering blood sugar levels.

There are three types of soluble fiber supplements: psyllium, methylcellulose, and polycarbophil. Each has varying uses, side effects, and properties. Check with your doctor for dosage and other information.

No matter what type of fiber supplement you decide to take, follow these general guidelines:

- Drink at least 8 ounces of water with a serving of a fiber supplement.
- Check your blood sugar more often when adding fiber supplements.
- Check with your doctor to determine which medications you might need to take within 2 hours of consuming a fiber supplement.

TO YOUR HEALTH

Fiber food sources and supplements come in bulk or prepackaged containers. Buying in bulk is generally less expensive. Bulk supplements also tend to have fewer additives, and are often available at your local grocery store or online.

Spices

Two common spices that can help decrease blood sugar are fenugreek and cinnamon. Other spices that may also benefit diabetes by protecting against inflammation include turmeric, oregano, marjoram, and sage.

Fenugreek

The high fiber content of fenugreek helps delay gastric (stomach) emptying and decreases carbohydrate absorption. In addition, the seeds contain an amino acid that can boost the release of insulin. Adjustment of blood sugar–lowering medication is often necessary when using fenugreek. Work with your health-care team if you plan on using fenugreek on a regular basis.

Eating too much fenugreek can cause gas, bloating, and diarrhea. If you decide to try fenugreek, start slowly and build up gradually.

To help reduce blood sugar and cholesterol, use 5 grams (about ½ tablespoon) to 12 grams (about 1 tablespoon) of fenugreek seed per meal. Monitor your blood sugar afterward to see how you are affected.

Cinnamon

Cinnamon appears to have an insulin-like effect. Even though there are conflicting results in some studies, most of the studies show improved blood sugar when consuming cinnamon. The dosages used in these studies were between 1 and 6 grams of cinnamon a day. All of these doses were effective, but only participants who had taken the smallest amount of cinnamon (1 gram) continued to have improved blood glucose levels 20 days after they stopped taking it.

 RED FLAG

Too much cinnamon may be harmful. It contains a moderately toxic component called coumarin. Too much coumarin can cause liver and kidney damage.

The suggested doses of cinnamon are between 1 and 6 grams. Taking cinnamon at these doses appears to have no adverse effects. One gram of cinnamon is about ⅕ teaspoon, 3 grams is ½ teaspoon, and 6 grams is a little more than a teaspoon. If you decide to take cinnamon to help control blood sugar, check with your doctor first.

Anti-Inflammatory and Antioxidant Supplements

Diabetics and prediabetics are prone to more inflammation and consequently more advanced glycation end-products (AGEs). AGEs are chemical reactions from sugars and proteins in the body that naturally occur with aging. Starting from infancy, AGEs form at a slow rate in the normal body, but become accelerated with more available glucose.

AGEs can be compared to a process of caramelization that occurs when cooking foods. AGEs happen internally, resulting in tough, damaged tissue. To help stabilize the AGEs process, antioxidants and anti-inflammatory supplements and foods can be helpful for people with diabetes.

Omega-3 Fatty Acids

Omega-3 fats can decrease inflammation, lower triglyceride levels, and may even help prevent insulin resistance. There are three types of omega-3 fatty acids: alpha linolenic acid (ALA), eicosapentaenoic acid (EPA), and docosahexanenoic acid (DHA).

EPA and DHA fatty acids are the active form of the omega-3 fatty acids and are the easiest to absorb. Food sources high in EPA and DHA are fatty fish, such as salmon, mackerel, albacore tuna, Atlantic herring, and sardines. ALA acid is found in vegetable oil, and seeds and nuts such as flax and chia seeds and walnuts. However, when consumed in this form the body needs to convert it into EPA and DHA (active forms). Aging, health variations, and individual differences influence our ability to convert ALA into EPA and DHA. Consequently, taking omega-3 fatty acids from fish oil supplements and fish is recommended.

The recommended omega-3 fatty acid supplement is 1,000 to 2,000 milligrams per day. Prior to taking this supplement, check with your pharmacist or your doctor to see if it can interact with any of your medications.

CoQ10

CoQ10 is a vitamin-like substance that acts as a strong antioxidant. It is normally produced by the body, but its production can be impaired in some cases by metabolic disorders.

Preliminary evidence indicates that taking CoQ10 twice a day may help to improve blood pressure and to slow the AGEs process. It may also be effective for people with congestive heart failure. The studies show that it can reduce symptoms of heart failure, such as shortness of breath and swelling, and can help provide energy to cells.

CoQ10 is fat soluble, so take it with foods containing fat, such as nuts or avocado, for better absorption. It is manufactured from beets and sugar cane with specific strains of yeast and is found naturally in foods such as seafood, poultry, pork, and beef. CoQ10 has no known side effects.

The recommended dose is between 75 and 200 milligrams per day. Dosing can vary depending on the condition it is being used for; check with your doctor.

Vitamin C

Vitamin C (ascorbic acid) is a highly effective antioxidant; even small amounts can protect the body from damage done by AGEs and exposure to toxins and pollutants. Studies have shown that taking 300 milligrams a day can significantly decrease the risk of death from coronary heart disease.

Foods high in vitamin C include sweet red and green peppers, citrus fruits and juices, and strawberries. For best consumption of vitamin C, eat foods like peppers, cabbage, and tomatoes raw. Cooking foods high in vitamin C will destroy much of this nutrient.

Since vitamin C is water soluble, divide doses evenly throughout the day and use no more than 1,000 milligrams a day. Dividing the doses is helpful because water-soluble vitamins are flushed out of the body through urination within a couple of hours after eating them.

Vitamin E

Vitamin E helps prevent oxidative stress to the body. Studies using large doses of vitamin E (under 400 IU) have shown some negative results, whereas lower doses have shown positive results. It may be that in high doses, vitamin E causes an imbalance in other antioxidants. Dietary antioxidants such as vitamin C and E, carotenoids, and flavonoids all work together in a synergistic way.

Vitamin E is a fat-soluble vitamin, so it can be stored in the liver and used as needed. Good sources include sunflower seeds, wheat germ, and almonds.

The recommended dosage to help with AGEs is 20 to 400 IU a day. The recommended daily allowance recommended by the National Institutes of Health is 15 IU a day. The tolerable upper limit for vitamin E recommended by the United States Institute of Medicine is 1,500 IU.

Overeating and AGEs

If you are overweight, you will have more AGEs and inflammation. Just by eating less, you can help prevent AGEs and inflammation. Other preventive ways to decrease the progression of AGE is to eat a diet high in antioxidants and lose weight if you are overweight.

Some supplements and foods may help with weight management. *Thermogenesis* is the production of heat by cells. It can be induced immediately by exercise, shivering, and simply by eating. With exercise, thermogenesis is increased more in people with more muscle mass because muscle tissue burns more calories than fat tissue.

> **DEFINITION**
>
> **Thermogenesis** refers to heat production, which uses up calories. The body naturally produces heat to keep all the organs functioning properly. Some outside forces, such as exercise and eating, will increase heat production in the body.

Eating hot, spicy foods such as chili peppers and ginger root, or consuming foods that contain catechin and caffeine, can increase thermogenesis. Catechin is a naturally occurring phenol in some plant foods like green teas and chili peppers that acts as an antioxidant and thermogenic enhancer. Thermogenesis by food consumption only lasts for a couple of hours, so it may be helpful to consume some of these foods in small amounts throughout the day.

Green tea is a thermogenic beverage that can promote fat burning, especially if used in small amounts throughout the day. In addition to being thermogenic, it contains a relaxing agent called L-theanine. Theanine can help reduce stress as well as improve thinking and mood. Since green tea contains caffeine, it is best to stop drinking it about 4 to 6 hours before bedtime. For best effectiveness, use plain green hot or iced tea, not the sugary beverages called green tea and sold in bottles.

Green tea is sold in supplemental pill form, but it is not known if this has the same effect as drinking the tea. For a thermogenic benefit, drink up to 3 cups of a strongly brewed tea every day. You also get a benefit from lightly brewed tea.

Special Beverages, Condiments, and Foods

Donna and Caran and their husbands, Scott and Adam, are going on a one-week camping trip in an RV they rented. Donna and Caran are planning the food.

Caran called Donna. "Hi, Donna, are you ready for our big camping trip?" she asked.

Donna half-heartedly replied, "No, not really." She paused, and then said, "I'm trying to eat well to keep my blood sugar in control and I'm also trying to lose a little weight. It's been easy at home with the conveniences of a kitchen, but I'm a little worried about trying to eat right while camping. The only refrigeration we'll have is a couple of coolers and the only way to cook will be with a kerosene stove or an open fire."

Caran said, "Yeah, I know what you mean, but maybe we can arrange to take some healthy foods that don't need refrigeration or cooking." She thought for a minute, and then added, "What if we take some low-carb tortillas, bottled water, and diet soda? Those things don't need constant refrigeration and we can get ice at the ranger's station for the water and soda."

"That sounds great!" Donna cheerfully replied. "Come to think of it, I can bring some packaged diabetic protein bars and canned shakes, too. They won't need refrigeration."

"Good idea. Let's also bring some apples, oranges, and potatoes. And some dried fruits, vegetables, and nuts, too, along with coffee and the usual condiments like salt and pepper packets and sugar substitutes. Are we missing anything?" asked Caran.

Donna thought for moment and said, "The guys are going to want a couple of beers during the week, but it shouldn't be a problem for us—neither of us likes beer and besides, it's high in calories."

Just in case you get in a pinch, diabetic shakes, bars, and low-carbohydrate tortillas can be helpful. However, what about using the sugar substitutes, salt, diet soda, alcohol, and coffee?

What About Alcohol?

Many people with diabetes know how foods affect their blood sugar, but are not sure about what alcohol can do. The American Diabetes Association (ADA) recommends you check with your health care provider before drinking alcohol. In small amounts (1 to 2 drinks per day), alcohol may help control blood pressure and heart disease, but in larger quantities it can cause havoc with your blood sugar and increase your blood pressure and triglyceride levels. To avoid complications with alcohol, limit your intake. If you are a woman, limit yourself to one drink per day, if you are a man, limit yourself to two drinks. One drink equals the following amounts of different types of alcohol:

- 5 oz. wine
- 12 oz. regular beer
- 3 oz. sherry or port
- 1 oz. hard liquor such as vodka, gin, or rum

If you choose to drink alcohol, wine may be the best choice since it contains flavonoids called resveratrol that can help decrease inflammation.

Alcohol with Insulin

If you use insulin or insulin-lowering medication, alcohol consumption will increase your risk of having a low blood sugar. Alcohol reduces glucose production by the liver and decreases the body's ability to release sugar into the blood. In addition, even small amounts of alcohol can decrease your ability to detect a low blood sugar and this decreased awareness is due to having a low blood sugar, not from the alcohol itself.

 RED FLAG

Don't drink on an empty stomach. To prevent low blood sugar, drink alcohol with a meal or snack that contains carbohydrates such as chips, crackers, fruit, yogurt, or bread.

Don't Drink Alcohol When ...

Don't drink alcohol if you have a fatty liver, high triglycerides, pancreatitis, cirrhosis, hepatitis, or advanced neuropathy. Even small amounts of alcohol can exacerbate these conditions. You might also want to avoid alcohol if you want to lose weight. Each gram of alcohol has 7 calories, and so one shot (1½ oz.) of vodka has about 124 calories.

How Many Carbohydrates?

Hard liquors like vodka have no carbohydrates, but some alcohol drinks, like beer and wine, do. Even though it helps to have some carbohydrates with alcohol, too many is not desirable either. They can contribute to an elevated blood sugar. Carbohydrate contents of alcoholic drinks vary widely, so for specific carbohydrate gram content, check the label.

The carbohydrates in wine can vary depending on whether the wine is considered "dry" or "sweet." A 5 oz. glass of dry wine has only 3 grams of carbohydrates and 100 calories, but a 5 oz. glass of sweeter dessert wine has 15 grams of carbohydrates and 165 calories.

Sugar Substitutes

People often ask about sugar substitutes; many people worry that artificial and even natural sweeteners are not healthy. Extensive research has shown that this is not true. Low-calorie and calorie-free sweeteners are considered safe and are supported by the American Diabetes Association, American Dental Association, and the American Cancer Society.

Studies have shown that sugar substitutes are not only safe, but that when used in the diet to replace added sugars, they help regulate body weight. Use a small amount of sugar substitute to enhance palatability and to adhere to a lower-calorie diet. Too much can interfere with the natural flavor of foods and possibly cause food sensitivity.

If you suspect you have particular sugar substitute sensitivity, avoid the suspected sweetener. If desired, try another low or non-caloric sweetener. According to food allergy specialists, a food intolerance may be prevented by not overdoing any one food or food additive. This includes artificial sweeteners.

Noncaloric Sweetener Guidelines

Common non-nutritive sweeteners approved by the U.S. Food and Drug Administration (FDA) include aspartame (Equal), saccharine (Sweet'N Low), and sucralose (Splenda, Neotame, and Stevia). Studies done by cancer researchers found that an acceptable daily intake for aspartame is about 50 mg/kg per day; for saccharine, about 15 mg/kg per day; and for sucralose, about 5 mg/kg per day.

Sugar Alcohols

One new sweetener that was approved in 2007 is Truvia. It is a combination of Stevia and erythritol, a sugar alcohol. Sugar alcohols occur naturally in plants and contain minimal calories. A drawback, however, is that they are not as sweet as sugar (sucrose), so a larger quantity is required to obtain the same amount of sweetness. Some people may experience gastrointestinal upset after eating too much sugar alcohol.

Amounts of up to 20 grams per day have been found to be well tolerated in most individuals. Everyone is different, so use sugar alcohol based on your tolerance level.

Diet Soda

Drinking diet soda will not, as a rule, raise your blood sugar. However, if more than one can at a time is consumed, it could have an effect on some diabetic individuals because of the caffeine content. Caffeine consumptions of 90 to 400 milligrams per serving can increase blood sugar about 2 to 8 percent. One 12-ounce can of Diet Mountain Dew has 55 milligrams of caffeine, while a 12-ounce can of diet Coke has 45 milligrams. Drinking the equivalent of two cans or more may cause an increase in blood sugar.

Recently, there have been numerous news stories about soft drinks and weight gain. The studies concerning this have shown that people who drink two or more cans of diet soda in a day were more likely to gain weight. These studies were observational and it is impossible to know what really causes an effect. Perhaps people with a very poor diet drink more diet sodas, or maybe the diet soda drinkers in the study switched to diet when they started gaining weight. Further, what about the many individuals who have been thin most of their lives and drink a can or two of diet soda every day? It appears that there are still a lot of unanswered questions, but having one can of diet soda a day along with a healthy diet is not a problem.

Coffee

Research from several studies shows that people who drink one to three cups of coffee a day have a decreased risk of acquiring diabetes and preventing the progression of prediabetes into type 2 diabetes. While both decaffeinated and regular coffee appear to decrease the risk, regular coffee seems to work better. In the studies, people who drank only decaffeinated coffee showed only half the reduction for diabetes risk as people who drank coffee with caffeine.

This can be a little confusing since caffeine can increase the blood sugar slightly, but for people who do not already have diabetes, it is effective. The reason might be related to the components that make up coffee.

In a study reported in 2011, researchers examined three components in coffee: caffeic acid, caffeine, and chlorogenic acid. They discovered that all three components may inhibit the activity of the toxic processes that can cause type 2 diabetes:

- Caffeic acid had the strongest protective effect of the three. It is an antioxidant that can enhance the immune system as well as act as anti-inflammatory agent for the body.

- Chlorogenic acid in coffee is a known antioxidant that slows the release of glucose into the bloodstream after a meal and helps prevent liver glycogen from turning into glucose.

- Caffeine, which has a bitter-tasting quality, is a stimulant. There is strong scientific evidence that caffeine in coffee improves mood, exercise performance, and breathing disorders.

If you find that caffeine increases your blood sugar but you want to drink coffee for its other benefits, try using decaffeinated or a lower-caffeinated coffee. Dark-roasted coffees have slightly less caffeine than the lighter roasts. The roasting process reduces the bean's caffeine content, and at the same time increases the anti-oxidant components. Both the American Medical Association and the American Cancer Society have endorsed the safety of moderate caffeine consumption.

> **TO YOUR HEALTH**
>
> If you decide to drink coffee, use coffee creamers and sugar sparingly—or avoid adding them altogether and drink your coffee black.

The caffeine in coffee and tea is not a threat to overall blood pressure problems. Caffeine may raise blood pressure slightly, but this has been shown to be only temporary without long-term effects. However, individuals who are sensitive to too much caffeine will still need to monitor their intake. Some of the reasons for the sensitivity include having anxiety, using certain types of medications, and having some types of heart arrhythmias.

How Much Salt?

Since diabetes puts you at high risk for cardiovascular disease and elevated blood pressure, your sodium intake should only be between 1,500 and 2,000 milligrams a day. The amount of sodium you eat can add up in a hurry, even if you don't use the salt shaker. If you do, keep in mind that salt itself contains 2,325 milligrams of sodium per teaspoon.

If you are like most people, you will probably take in most of your sodium in the food you eat. Some foods can increase your intake of sodium to over 1,000 milligrams with just a single serving. One 5-gram bouillon cube, for example, has 1,200 milligrams of sodium. Even a $1/2$ cup of 2 percent cottage cheese has 460 milligrams of sodium. Be sure to read the food labels to see how much sodium you're getting in a serving. (See Chapter 6 for more about reading food labels.)

More Potassium and Magnesium, Less Sodium

To lower sodium in your diet, eat more fresh fruits and vegetables and whole unprocessed foods. In addition to being lower in sodium, this type of diet is usually higher in potassium and magnesium.

Potassium is essential to our health. It helps heart and other muscles contract, lowers blood pressure, and regulates fluid and minerals. Excess amounts are excreted in the urine. To obtain adequate potassium in your diet, include foods like sweet potatoes, yogurt, apricots, and spinach.

A diet high in magnesium helps regulate blood pressure and blood glucose levels, and also helps maintain normal muscle and nerve function. The minimum daily allowance for magnesium is 400 milligrams a day. To obtain adequate magnesium in your diet, include foods like bran cereals, pumpkin seeds, spinach, almonds, artichokes, dried beans, and fish.

Diabetic Specialty Products

Diabetic specialty foods include a variety of products such as nutritionals, low-carbohydrate breads and pasta, snacks, and sugar-free desserts and candy. At times some of these foods can be helpful and convenient to use, but they are not essential to a healthy diet and they can be expensive.

Many of these products contain a reduced amount of added sugars and carbohydrate and are often sweetened with a sugar alcohol and/or artificial sweetener. Some also contain added fiber and protein, which can be helpful for satiety and blood sugar control. You might also want to check the ingredient list for other less desirable ingredients.

For best quality, always look for whole unprocessed ingredients such as flax meal and whole grains, and do not use anything with partially hydrogenated vegetables oils. They are trans-fats and are five times worse for you than saturated fats. They can both raise your "bad" cholesterol and decrease your "good" cholesterol.

In addition to avoiding the trans-fats, minimize other less desirable ingredients:

- High fructose corn syrup (HFCS): Especially if listed as one of the first three ingredients
- Syrup (any type): Especially if listed as one of the first three ingredients
- Monosodium glutamate (MSG): Avoid if sensitive; common reactions include headaches, rashes, and nausea
- Sodium nitrite and sodium nitrate: Strong cancer risk association
- Refined flours: If listed as one of the first three ingredients
- Sugar: Especially if listed as one of the first three ingredients
- Cornstarch: If listed as one of the first three ingredients

Common ingredients on food labels that can sound foreign or even scary, but which are nutritious include:

- **Vitamins:** Pyridoxine hydrochloride (vitamin B-6), folate (folic acid B vitamin), riboflavin (vitamin B-2), thiamine (vitamin B-1), cobalamin (vitamin B-12), niacinamide (vitamin B-3), choline (B vitamin), biotin (B vitamin), ascorbic acid (vitamin C), and cholecalciferol (vitamin D3)
- **Minerals:** Potassium chloride, potassium iodide, potassium chloride, potassium citrate, manganese sulfate, magnesium phosphate, sodium citrate, ferrous sulfate (iron), calcium phosphate, chromium picolinate
- **Fatty acids:** Soy lecithin, canola oil, olive oil, soy oil, omega-3 fatty acids

- **Fibers:** Cellulose, inulin, lignin, waxes, chitins, pectins, beta-glucans, oligosaccharides, wheat bran, corn bran, psyllium, guar gum, bean gums, xanthan gum
- **Proteins:** Soy isolates, milk protein such as caseins, whey, glutamine, egg white

Nutritionals

A nutritional is a food product with added vitamins, minerals, fiber, or amino acids that replace all or part of a meal. Common diabetic nutritionals include Extend and Glucerna products. Even though these products can cost a little more, convenience is their selling point.

Extend and Glucerna nutritionals come in bars, shakes, and miscellaneous snacks. These products use a combination of protein, fat, and complex lower-glycemic carbohydrates that can help control blood sugar for a longer time.

Low-Carbohydrate Breads and Pasta

Many of the breads that are low in carbohydrate are also higher in protein and fiber. The types of protein commonly used in these products include soy or gluten (wheat protein). Fibers most commonly used include cellulose, wheat bran, corn bran, and oat fiber. Many of these products can help with satiety because both protein and fiber can help slow down carbohydrate absorption.

Low-Carbohydrate Desserts and Candy

Many companies now manufacture lower-carbohydrate desserts and candy. The usual sugar-free puddings and cookies can be found in most grocery stores. Although these products can be tasty, they contain a lot of refined ingredients and calories without a lot of vitamins, minerals, or fiber. Some may also cause gastrointestinal discomfort due to sugar alcohols. Save these foods for once-in-awhile treats only.

Resources

To learn more about how to manage your diabetes, the following books and websites are good places to start.

Books

- Beale, Lucy, Joan Clark, and Barbara Forsberg. *The Complete Idiot's Guide to Terrific Diabetic Meals.* Indianapolis, IN: Alpha Books, 2004.

- Beale, Lucy, and Joan Clark-Warner. *The Complete Idiot's Guide Glycemic Index Cookbook.* Indianapolis, IN: Alpha Books, 2009.

- ———. *The Complete Idiot's Guide to Glycemic Index Weight Loss, Second Edition.* Indianapolis, IN: Alpha Books, 2010.

- Beale, Lucy, and Sandy Couvillon. *The Complete Idiot's Guide to Low-Carb Meals, Second Edition.* Indianapolis, IN: Alpha Books, 2012.

- Brand-Miller, Jennie, Kaye Foster-Powell, and Philippa Sandall. *The New Glucose Revolution: Low GI Eating Made Easy.* Cambridge, MA: Da Capo Press, 2005.

Websites

American Association of Clinical Endocrinologists (AACE)
www.aace.com

American Association of Diabetes Educators (AADE)
www.diabeteseducator.org

American Diabetes Association (ADA)
www.diabetes.org

Choose MyPlate.gov
choosemyplate.gov/myplate/index.aspx

Meal Planning Made Simple
mealsmatter.org/

Monthly Meal Planner
monthlymealplanner.com/

National Diabetes Information Clearinghouse (NIDDK)
diabetes.niddk.nih.gov

Natural Standard Database—An Authority on Integrative
Medicine
naturalstandard.com

Index